Nursing: Your Registration
The Guide to Revalidation with Ease

To Alex
Best wishes in your
continuing development
lovely to meet you at
RCN Congress 2022

Claire Picton

Claire Picton

First published 2016

Copyright © Claire Picton 2016

The moral right of the author has been asserted.

All rights reserved. No part of this work may be reproduced or stored in an informational retrieval system, without the express permission of the publisher in writing.

ISBN 978-1534691155

Published by:
10-10-10 Publishing
Markham, ON
Canada

Disclaimer note:

This book must be used in conjunction with the Nursing and Midwifery Council's guidance on revalidation: normally found on the NMC revalidation microsite. The author accepts no responsibility for nurses' failure to successfully re-register with the Nursing and Midwifery Council, for England, Wales, Scotland and Northern Ireland.

In memory of
Alex Bell (neé Arnold) 1953 To 2015.
Alex was a joyful, generous, loving person and friend, in addition to being an enthusiastic, caring and effective nurse. She would have loved Damsels in Success and been thrilled to be involved with this book.
With thanks to
Francesca and Laurence Bell
Young people who she was the proud mother of.

With love to
My mother, Phyllis Cook; my husband, Ken Buckler and our son Jay Buckler-Picton; my long-standing friend (almost sister!) Rachel Robinson. They all deserve huge thanks for loving and supporting me and for enduring my procrastination!

Contents

Acknowledgements	vii
Foreword	ix
If you read nothing else, read this!	xi
Chapter 1: What is revalidation about?	1
Chapter 2: Taking personal responsibility for your revalidation	17
Chapter 3: Planning your future career development	33
Chapter 4: Daily work and revalidation	45
Chapter 5: Will the registered nurse step up and shine please?	61
Chapter 6: The art and science within the registered nurse	75
Chapter 7: The reflective registered nurse	85
Chapter 8: Owning your portfolio	99
Chapter 9: Removing drama from the lives of registered nurses	113
Chapter 10: Trusting others, trusting yourself	125
Summary	137
About the author	139

Acknowledgements

Many people in both my private and professional life have helped me. Some I have known for most of my life, others I met fleetingly but had a profound effect on me. I am sorry that there is not space to name them all here, since I am grateful to every one of them.

Debs Addley, Juliet Anderson, Jayne Austin, Jan Bell, Marie Buckler, Denise Chaffer, Lyn Crouchman, Juliet Irwin, Soline Jerram, Sue Leddington, Maggie Lord, Mary Murcott, Noreen Rice, Liz Smith, Sharon Smith, Wendy Stevens, Sue West, are just a few of the many nurses who over the years have supported and nurtured me.

The members and staff of RCN London region, RCN Outer North West London and RCN Chichester Branches deserve thanks for the opportunities that they gave me. The members of the Emergency Nurse Consultants Association and the Royal College of Nursing (RCN) Emergency Care Association for support in a changing environment. All the nurses that I have worked with over the years, and those I currently do, have enriched my life. Thanks also to Sister Jennifer at St Mary's Convent & Nursing Home for offering me an unexpected opportunity and generous support.

Claire Picton

The following are just a small number of people who influence and support nurses nationally and I have been fortunate enough to meet - Cecilia Anim, Professor Viv Bennett, Joanne Bosanquet, Michael Brown, Peter Carter, Professor Jane Cummings, Janet Davies, Stuart MacKenzie, Rod Thompson, Jason Warriner.

Thanks to all the staff at RCNi, particularly Nick Lipley, Graham Scott, Helen Hyland and Sandra Lynch, who supported me when I was Editor of Emergency Nurse Journal.

Lucie Bradbury and the Damsels in Success Directors have inspired me, challenged me, supported me and helped me keep myself accountable.

David Picton took on the role of dad and introduced me to cars and steam trains. Giving me the Pioneer nameplate gave me something to aspire to.

As a Christian, I have to thank God for putting all these people in my life and for the love, faith and charity He has provided for me.

Without patients and their precious ones there would be no job for healthcare professionals. I am hugely indebted to those who have allowed me to care for them, when they probably would rather have not met me in the circumstances that they did!

Foreword

I am pleased to recommend this book as essential reading for all nurses and midwives in the UK as they prepare for revalidation of their professional registration.

Claire's knowledge and expertise are a distillation of her extensive career in Higher Education, as a Nurse Consultant in Emergency Care and past Editor of the Emergency Nurse Journal. This book is likely to be one that you will want to keep referring back to.

Within the book the information builds on the guidance from the Nursing and Midwifery Council (NMC) and it includes exercises to get you started or make you think differently. Taking the first step can be the hardest, so Claire writes with encouragement and exhorts you to have a 'can do' attitude, providing you with tools to commence; then to easily and successfully achieve your revalidation process.

This book aims to assist those who are in clinical practice, managers or educators in their varying needs for revalidation. Whichever field or role you work in, whether you are just revalidating or are doing both revalidation and confirming, this book will help you and also point you to further resources. It:

Claire Picton

- demonstrates various ways to collect evidence.
- shows how to consider your self-care, to aid you in caring for people that you encounter in your work.
- will benefit you in your ongoing journey of self-discovery.

Continuing Professional Development (CPD) linked with the NMC (2015) Code of Conduct is a key aspect of revalidation and this book guides you along that path.

Reflective writing is also a significant component of revalidation. In the first year alone there are likely to be 3 million reflections which, as Charlotte McArdle, Chief Nursing Officer for Northern Ireland, stated at the Florence Nightingale Foundation Annual Conference in March 2016 that is "3 million opportunities for practice improvement". The key tenets of the NMC (2015) Code of Conduct are to prioritise people, practise effectively, preserve safety, and promote professionalism and trust. These are examined as applied to the nurse, or midwife, in addition to end users.

This book is a very helpful and useful guide on your journey and will be a helpful addition to your reading list.

Professor Elizabeth Robb, OBE.
Chief Executive.
The Florence Nightingale Foundation, UK.

If you read nothing else – read this!

The emphasis in this book is that revalidation of your nurse registration starts and ends with you, the reader. This is made clear and explicit in the first part of the title – 'Nursing: Your Registration'. This book unashamedly focuses on you and I have referred to the Code of Conduct (NMC, 2015) in addition to using values devised by Bradbury (2013). These values are that we need to: fill ourselves up first; take personal responsibility and look inward; let go of control and trust; embrace our imperfections and shine; bring love and light to every situation; not get caught up in drama; use the best masculine systems to stay in our feminine flow; encourage not judge; ask for help and receive it. These are intended to assist you to achieve success with ease. I believe these are applicable to everyone, although I acknowledge they were devised for women (90% of nurses are women).

The key part is that you, the reader, have to take action and responsibility. Without this engagement, there is little or no chance of success. The first thing towards revalidation is to make a start and glean as much information as possible - you have done that by reading this introduction. Well done! Congratulate yourself. The world needs nurses and it needs you to remain a nurse.

Claire Picton

It is easier to accomplish and enjoy reaching your prize with a partner, peer or guide, although some nurses will successfully revalidate with minimal aid. As an author, I can assist you with my guidance: I can share my knowledge and experience; I can direct you to resources (NMC, 2016a) and I can suggest how you can achieve revalidation with ease.

This book was conceived because I value my nursing colleagues and want to support you. I have witnessed in clinical practice how worried and anxious the mere word 'revalidation' has made many nurses. Even though it is only about continuing professional development and an extension of the renewal process that has been in place since the 1990s. My aim in writing this book is to; alleviate some of your concerns, help you to believe in yourself, encourage you to ask for help, and to stimulate you into taking action.

If, after reading this book, you are less anxious, less worried and/or you have taken positive and informed action to revalidate, then I will have achieved something worthwhile. I am keen to serve you and my website offers additional material that will be of benefit to you.

Point 9 (NMC, 2015) states that as a nurse I must "share (your) skills, knowledge and experience for the benefit of people receiving care and your colleagues". Therefore, this book is my gift to you and I hope as you unwrap it, it allows you to live in the present (since present also means gift) and attain your goal of revalidation.

Nursing: Your Registration

My hopes lie in you as the nurse of the future. Who knows, you may even be my nurse in the future.

Come with me and step into your journey…

With love and laughter
Claire

Bradbury L (Ed) (2013) The F Factor. CreateSpace Independent Publishing Platform.
NMC (2015) The Code of Conduct. NMC. London.

To continue travelling with my guidance go to: www.NurseRevalidationBook.co.uk

Chapter 1
What is revalidation about?

History of revalidation

It is useful to look back at events in history to have an idea of the reason why revalidation has arisen. History can also assist in preventing us making mistakes that have already occurred/been made by others. The organisations that have governed nursing registration have changed over the years. Nurse registration is a relatively new concept, which commenced in the 20th century, and one that was hard-won.

Brief overview of registration and re-registration	
General Nursing Council (GNC)	Created in December 1919.
	Nurse Registration commenced in 1921.
	Dis-established in July 1983. Trust created.
UK Central Council for Nursing & Midwifery (UKCC)	Created in 1983.
Post-Registration Education and Practice Project (PREPP)	Was developed in the late eighties.
Post-Registration Education and Practice (PREP)	Established in 1990 and revalidation is built on its framework.
Nursing & Midwifery Council (NMC)	Formed in 2002
Revalidation of Nurse Registration.	Piloted in 2014
	Commenced in April 2016.

Table 1

Claire Picton

Many employers asked nurses to bring their PREP portfolio, with evidence of their continuing professional development, to their yearly personal development review (PDR). In the NHS with Agenda for Change it was often a requirement. However, if the nurse did not do this, it was only up to the employer to take action. The UKCC, nor NMC, did not make it a requirement that the nurse's portfolio had to be seen. Any registered nurse could be randomly selected to submit their PREP portfolio (3 years of evidence) to the UKCC, then the NMC, and would be bound to comply or risk losing their registration. This seldom occurred or only a very small number of registrants had to do this. There were less defined criteria about what needed to be in the portfolio as well.

The PREP aims were to ensure that nurses kept up to date and progress their development. Revalidation builds on this and assumes all nurses were already keeping a portfolio and undertaking continual professional development.

Within England, Agenda for change was introduced in 2004 (NHS, 2005) provided a positive development in terms of insisting that all staff keep a portfolio. It allowed for a more structured way of demonstrating updating and progression in one's chosen career, indicated by the Key Skills Framework (Department of Health, 2004). The difference between PREP & revalidation is that there is focus on the NMC Code of Conduct (NMC, 2015) and there is clear and detailed structure to the process. Although the nurse does not have to prove competence, they do have to show evidence to a 'confirmer' that they have undertaken the minimum number of hours in both clinical practice and study hours.

Previously, the renewal was only dependent on the registrant signing to say they were able to stay on the register as they had maintained their competence and they have completed the requisite number of clinical practice hours. There was no requirement for every nurse to discuss their reflections with anyone else nor to show their evidence of continuing professional development (CPD), unless the NMC asked to see it.

The confirmer role simply confirms that the nurse has undertaken the process required for revalidation. It will normally be your line manager, but there is guidance from the NMC about who else can be chosen. The confirmer is not required to judge whether the nurse is competent. (NMC, 2016a)

There has been an emphasis on protecting the public following the Francis report (2013). The focus of revalidation is protecting the public. It is worth recalling the basic tenet (idea) of nurse registration has always been to protect the public. It does also protect your personal nurse registration, providing you do not do, or omit to do, anything that jeopardises it.

The NMC (2016a) and Department of Health have decreed that from April 2016 nurses will have to re-register using the new revalidation process. It allows nurses to evidence their continuing improvement of their practice to assure the public has confidence in practicing nurses. The value that fits with this is that we have to let go of control and trust (Bradbury, 2013) since the NMC are our governing body.

Purpose of revalidation

Revalidation is about nurses remaining on the NMC register. Being a nurse is a professional role and registration is a legal requirement in order to practice as a nurse.

The Francis report (2013) highlighted mistakes in the checking and reporting of professionals' registration, as well as the numerous other issues that arose and were documented in the extremely long report that many nurses have perhaps not had an inclination to read in full. Revalidation purports to protect the public. It will only do so, providing nurses embrace the value of continuing professional development and recognise their personal responsibility in their progression. Otherwise there is a danger of revalidation becoming just a process that must be gone through. As professionals, nurses need to protect the public, but in order to do that they also need to protect themselves. By revalidating and thus maintaining their registration, nurses are putting themselves first, which is as it should be (Bradbury, 2013). Looking after yourself in order to get into the best physical, spiritual and mental state to care for other people well is vital and you will have to sign a 'Health and Character' declaration as part of your revalidation process. Additionally, Point 20.9 highlights the importance of caring for your own health (NMC, 2015) and this equates with 'filling ourselves up first' (Bradbury (2013).

The way revalidation will work best, is if the outcome is that each registered nurse learns and develops during the process and is committed to their own self-care to deliver the best care that they can to patients. Whether this is direct care or indirect care, which managers and educators are more likely to provide.

The best way to protect the public is not to have a tick-box exercise. The premise of this book is to assist registered nurses to become the best registered nurse that they can, with ease. This involves nurses embedding and appreciating the value of life-long learning in their daily practice.

Revalidation should be an opportunity for nurses to reflect on their progress, what they have learnt and be proud of their career development. It may also be a chance to prove knowledge and competence to themselves. As people commonly focus on the negatives, on mistakes that have been made and what has not been achieved this may be a chance for nurses to view their clinical practice and personal development in a positive manner (NMC, 2015). This may increase their morale, reduce stress and prevent burnout.

As many confirmers will be line managers, and probably a large number of those will be nurses as well, they will be keen to ensure that the nurses who work for them successfully revalidate. Otherwise it will have a negative impact on their workforce/team if nurses leave because they decide not to revalidate or are unable to for some reason. For nurses who are employed by an agency, it is still in the employers' best interest to assist them with revalidation – so ask how they will be doing this with you.

The public and revalidation

Although the NMC Code of Conduct has been present to guide the practice of registered nurses, it is unlikely that the majority of nurses have referred to it on a regular basis. As the NMC (2015) has decreed the Code of Conduct needs to be looked at when reflection occurs and the correct section picked, this will ensure that nurses will frequently refer to it in the future.

Use of the NMC (2015) Code of Conduct will become an integral part of revalidation. Nurses should consider how their daily clinical practice and their Code of Conduct link when they are working. Easy and visible access to the Code of Conduct in each nurses' place of work is advisable to facilitate this.

The role of the NMC is to protect the public, which is why they have developed a Code of Conduct that nurses must adhere to. This should provide clarity about their role for nurses and expectations of the general public about nurses.

The role of the confirmer is to understand the process for revalidation and to be studying the Code of Conduct whether they are a registered nurse or not (NMC, 2015).

The 4 parts of the Code of Conduct (NMC, 2015) are:

- Prioritise people.
- Practise effectively.
- Preserve safety.
- Promote professionalism and trust.

Each part of the Code of Conduct is further divided into sub-sections. Points 2.3 and 3.3, plus the paragraph about patients and service users on page 3, (NMC, 2015) seem particularly relevant to discussion about the public and revalidation.

The Code of Conduct (NMC, 2015) will be referred to frequently throughout this book. It should be referred to at least once a week, preferably daily, by all nurses.

- Prioritise people is ensuring that the people you nurse are put first and treated with respect, dignity and confidentiality, but that they also have a choice about their treatment.

- Practise effectively. This is where the continuing professional development fits in as the aim to use an evidence base for clinical practice. It is the responsibility, and always has been, of every registered nurse to develop themselves and keep up to date with changes in nursing practice. The new revalidation process simply sets out a more structured approach than the previous registration renewal. Some nurses will do the minimum and other nurses have already been doing a large amount of work to develop themselves.
- Preserving safety of themselves is crucial, also safety of others: those in your care, but also their loved ones and the general public.
- Nurses must promote professionalism and trust, they must uphold the Code of Conduct in their contact with people. (NMC, 2015.) For the majority of the sections of the Code the emphasis appears to be on others. However, I would suggest in order to serve others, you need to ensure that you look after yourself first. This is not a selfish act nor meant in an arrogant way, but in a way that puts you in the best physical, mental and social health/state so that you can give to others. (Bradbury, 2013)

The nurse and revalidation

Revalidation is non-negotiable so how can it be done with ease?

How can you make yourself feel excited about revalidation? Remember when you were studying to be a nurse and you looked forward to finding out about nursing? (Wicks, 2005) Reading what others had written about nursing enthused you. Talking to others who were studying with you. How can you make it fun or at least a pleasant experience? (Buzan & Buzan, 1995) Raise your vibration!

Revalidation will:

- Provide you with an opportunity to rekindle that excitement about being the registered nurse that you wanted to become.
- Give you an opportunity to review your career and positive progress so far.
- Allow you to see how much you have achieved.
- Allows you to feel confident about your ability to revalidate your nurse registration.

Planning is a key factor. What are your intentions with regard to revalidation? Are you intending to gather evidence, planning to attend courses/study days/teaching sessions across the 3 years? Do you know how you will achieve your intentions? Or will you continue to put everybody else first and then be rushing around in year 3 trying to achieve 3 years' worth of evidence? (Holt, 2012)

The 6Cs were proposed as "Our culture of compassionate care" in England (Cummings, 2012), but they can equally apply to nurses. Care, compassion, competence, communication, courage, commitment for ourselves to allow our self-development in order for us to then serve others. Self-care; compassion for you; obtaining competence; positive self-talk; courage to believe in yourself; commitment to do all the preceding things for yourself.

Reflection was a feature of PREP and has been retained in the revalidation process. There are specific minimum number of 5 reflective pieces that have to be completed over the 3 years and the prescribed forms must be used. (NMC, 2016a)

Time management is a skill that can be learnt and having a plan that works for you can be the key to success with ease. Do you need someone to help you be accountable for achieving your intentions? It can be easier to achieve with others. Telling others what you want or intend to attain plus a written plan sets out your expectations for yourself. (Redgrave & Townsend, 2005; Bradbury, 2013) See also Chapter 3.

Exercise 1.

	Some positive questions to ask oneself:	Some thoughts:
1.	What is the way I can do this with the least extra work for myself?	Everyone has busy lives, so it is about thinking smart, rather than working harder, to achieve what is necessary.
2.	How can I make revalidation benefit me as a nurse and a professional?	Focus on positive and negative aspects of work so that a healthy balance is seen. Positive feedback encourages and provides motivation.
3.	How can this improve my relationship with the people that I care for, in my nurse role?	Confidence in one's ability allows better delivery of care. The patients will feel safe being cared for by a confident and empathetic nurse.

As nurses, we serve others. How can we serve ourselves first? Do we believe that we deserve to do this? Self-care is vital (Richardson, 2009). What does service mean to you? (Bradbury, 2013)

Revalidation with ease

Some people have a clear idea of their purpose and have a detailed plan of how they wish their career to develop. If this is you, then you probably think you can skip this section. Although, you may read it and find just one thing you had not considered before. Alternatively, it could confirm that you are doing things in the correct way for you. If you are not clear on your purpose in life, then now is a great time to think about it. When you have answered the questions in the table on the next page, I suggest you put them into your portfolio.

What is my purpose, in relation to my role as a Registered Nurse?	What are my intentions, in relation to achieving my next revalidation?
Suggested questions to answer:	
When, where and how can I fulfil my purpose in life?	What date do I have to achieve my revalidation by?
	How much time do I have before my revalidation date?
Why am I a Registered Nurse?	
Why do I want to remain a Registered Nurse?	Who can assist me in my nursing career? And in achieving my intentions?
How do I achieve my revalidation?	Who will I choose to be my confirmer?
What is my responsibility in relation to revalidation of my registration?	Do you need a reflective discussion partner as well? If yes, who will you choose?
	What do I need to do?
What, why, when, how, where and who are good questions to be asking. (Kipling, 1969)	Where will I do it?
	When will I make a plan?
	How will I carry out my plan?
	How can it be done easefully?

Exercise 2

Why make life difficult for yourself? Many nurses do this. Often it is because they don't put themselves first and/or do not make carrying out their intentions their priority. Richardson (2009) and Bradbury (2013) have exercises that can help you in making your life easeful.

Planning is important and some guidance on making a plan, is available in Chapter 3 and on the website: www.NurseRevalidationBook.co.uk

How I got started

When I started my nurse training, it was based in a hospital School of Nursing and not at a University. The State Registered Nurse qualification was not rated at a particular level and I understood registration was 'for life'.

In my career, I have spent much time doing part-time study as I believe I am a professional and that I should grow and develop throughout my professional life.

Courses:	Length of study
'Post-registration' specialist Accident & Emergency Certificate	9 months
Diploma in Nursing	3 years
'Post-registration' Mentorship Certificate	6 months
BSc (Hons)	2 years
Masters in Nursing with Education [Practice Educator qualification]	3 years
Emergency Nurse Practitioner	1 semester
Sports Injury	1 semester

Table 2

In the 1970's there were two nursing journals, not today's abundance of journals, so researching information was simpler than processing all the information available now. Reading and discovering about nursing has always been important to me and enhances my credibility. I believe learning from experience and clinical practice is valuable. A useful guideline for my learning has been answering the "what, why, when, how, where and who questions?" (Kipling, 1969).

When the UKCC introduced PREP I thought about how to create my portfolio with relevant evidence but with the least amount of work, because I am realistic about how much time I have at my disposal. I could understand and value the importance of career progression and how keeping a portfolio linked with that. Moving to the revalidation process builds upon what I have been already doing for my continuing professional development.

Bradbury (2013) has values that resonate with me and I practice using them daily, with varying amounts of success. However, the more I practice the more easeful my life becomes.

My other achievement is this book and sharing my experience and knowledge that I have obtained over the last 40 years. If I can guide you through the process of revalidation, then it enables me to give back, because I have been fortunate to receive so much.

References:
Bradbury L (Ed) (2013) *The F Factor.* CreateSpace Independent Publishing Platform.
Buzan T & Buzan B (1995) *The Mind Map Book.* London. BBC Books.
Cummings J (2012) *Compassion in Practice. Nursing, midwifery and care staff. Our vision for the future.* London. Department of Health.
Department of Health (2004) *The Knowledge and Skills Framework (NHS KSF) and the Development Review Process.* London. Department of Health.

Francis R (2013) *Report of the Mid Staffordshire NHS Foundation Trust Public Inquiry Executive summary.* London. Department of Health.

Holt L (2012) *Get out of your own way. Stop sabotaging your business and learn to stand out in a crowded market.* London. National Alliance of Business Owners.

Kipling (1969) *The Elephant's Child.* London. Follett Publishing Company.

Kline N (2002) *Time to think. Listening to ignite the human mind.* London. Cassell.

NHS Employers (2005) *Agenda for Change. NHS Terms and Conditions Handbook.* London. Department of Health.

NMC (2015) *Revalidation. How to revalidate with the NMC. Requirements for renewing your registration.* London. NMC.

NMC (2016a) *Revalidation. How to revalidate with the NMC. Requirements for renewing your registration.* London. NMC.

Redgrave S & Townsend N (2005) *You can win at life! Unlock your potential and go for gold...* London. BBC Books.

Richardson C (2009) *The art of extreme self-care: transform your life one month at a time.* London. Hay House.

Wicks RJ (2005) *Overcoming secondary stress in medical and nursing practice: a guide to professional resilience and personal well-being.* Oxford. Oxford University Press.

www.NurseRevalidationBook.co.uk

Chapter 2
Taking personal responsibility for your revalidation

Achieving revalidation

Take personal responsibility as a professional is the starting point. It is therefore pertinent to ask - what is a professional?

Professionals value their skills, knowledge and expertise. Professionals practice their skills consistently to ensure they remain good at them. Professionals value and enjoy learning, thinking that it is good to acquire knowledge each day. Professionals want to become experts in at least one part of their job, if not in their whole job. It gives them satisfaction and a sense of self-worth.

Some have argued though that professionals serve themselves and being part of a professional body does not necessarily protect the public as the body wants to avoid the profession being brought into disrepute, rather than having a focus on protecting the public (Oakley, 1986). The NMC seems different as it states that its prime function is to protect the public (NMC, 2015).

I am entitled to call myself a Registered General Nurse only because I have qualified to do so and am registered with the NMC, the professional body for nurses and this is enshrined in law.

Will going through a revalidation process ensure that you will practice in a professional manner? It is your personal responsibility to:

- Maintain your knowledge so that it is current;
- Engage with the process and make it an authentic exercise;
- Have tangible outcomes that you have achieved and use them to demonstrate your learning;
- Be able to show staff who you work with that you are able to use your learning in your daily practice, ideally to the benefit of the people you work with.

What is personal responsibility? Each nurse has to believe that their registration and being a nurse professional is worth something to them. As in Chapter 1, exercise 2, where it was suggested you consider why you are a nurse and why you wish to remain one. The registration may be; worth retaining because it provides an income to support their family, of value because the role of a nurse is what they wish to retain, since they enjoy caring for people and providing help to them that only a nurse can.

My understanding is that professionals take personal responsibility and look inward. It is not about blaming other people, but looking at what you are thinking and doing as an individual that you have to own. Responsibility for asking for help (and knowing when we need to ask for help) and then taking responsibility to allow ourselves to receive that help, is part of team work and functioning as a health care professional. 'No-one is an island'. Connections are part of the human situation. (Bradbury, 2013.)

How to get started with revalidation

The key is to make a start, have courage and commit (Cummings, 2012), then just do it and you have. To continue, read the literature about revalidation and access the revalidation part of the NMC website. Ask for other nurses for help, found out what other nurses know and also speak with your confirmer. Ask your professional development department/team, if you have them in your workplace. If you pay a subscription to a union, commonly the Royal College of Nursing (RCN) or Unison, they both have a professional information resource. As a member make sure you access what they provide.

Successful people learn as much as they can about the topic they need to know about (Baretta, 2014) and there is plenty of information available. Discover as much about revalidation as you can. Well done for investing in this book as a start.

Building on the previous chapter, remember to take personal responsibility. It is your registration and therefore your responsibility to maintain it.

To find out your renewal date, visit the NMC online website (NMC, 2016a).

When you have registered and then logged in to your account, you will see a screen similar to the one below:

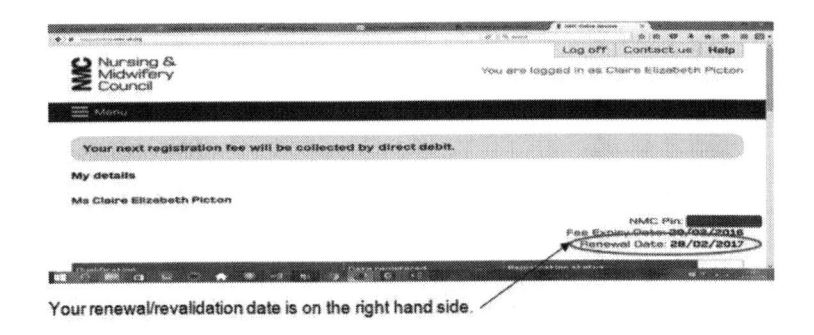

Your renewal/revalidation date is on the right hand side.

Your last date that you signed your declaration will have been 3 years before your revalidation date. So I last renewed on 28/02/2014, all my evidence between 2014 and 2017 is applicable. Though I have to relate it to the new revalidation process.

Plan and set intentions that you will be able to achieve and ask friends, family, work colleagues to assist you in keeping yourself accountable and on track. That means setting dates, but don't be hard on yourself if you are unable to keep them – it is only a setback. Consider the reasons why. If it was because you were busy with other people's needs, then you have to put yourself first. Do set new dates and promise yourself you will meet them. You probably don't break promises you make to other people, so why break promises you make to yourself? You are the most important asset in your life and therefore you must invest in yourself.

Calculate how many weeks you have until two months (60 days) before your revalidation. Then work out what you need to do and how you might achieve it. Planning to complete actions over a long period avoids having to rush around at the last minute, as that would be likely to make you feel stressed and overwhelmed. It may also make it unachievable in such a short period of time.

Table 3. An example plan

Month	To be achieved Examples:	How to achieve Examples:	Completed Yes No
January	Shadow a nurse who holds a more senior role than you.	Speak with or e-mail the person to ask if possible. Schedule agreed date in diary. Write objectives to be met on the day & share. Write reflection on shadow	
February	Read 2 articles.	Record the reference & a summary of each article. Share the above with staff in your area. Write to the journal about whether the article has helped your daily work.	
March	Write a piece of reflection about an aspect of your work.	Use NMC reflection outline. Pick a positive aspect of your work. Choose the model of reflection that seems most appropriate to you. Do not use the person's real name or any other identifying factors.	
April	Attend a meeting at work.	Photocopy the minutes of the meeting that show you were present. Write brief notes about how the meeting will help in your future practice.	

File all the above in your portfolio. Use NMC (2016a) forms, if appropriate.

Finding time, making time

This section considers time management. What can you realistically achieve in your place of work? 15 minutes of participatory study time a week should be achievable. Discuss with the staff who you work with about how you might do this.

Consider what resources you have in your place of work and how best to use the time accessing them. Is the Code of Conduct (NMC, 2015) easily accessible in your workplace?

As plans at work are often interrupted; by patients needing care that cannot be delayed, by students who require immediate support, and by reports that have to be given priority. It is much better to schedule 15 to 30 minutes each time you work, to achieve some participatory discussion, than an hour or more weekly or monthly. In my experience, the likelihood of the longer sessions happening is remote.

In your personal life. What are the absolute musts that you cannot delegate or request someone else to do or help you with? (Redgrave & Townsend, 2005)

Table 4. Example Week planner			
Day	Other (Self-care, etc)	Personal Life	Work
Monday	Listening to music, dancing, using foot spa, exercising.	Transporting a family member somewhere.	A busy day with high workload.
Tuesday	Swimming.	Internet grocery shopping.	15 minutes non-participatory study.
Wednesday	Bell-ringing.		15 minutes feedback recording.
Thursday	Watch 1 TV programme	Supporting a family member with studying.	15 minutes participatory study.
Friday	Exercising.		
Saturday	Visit friends.	Telephone a family member elsewhere.	
Sunday	Attend church service.		

Referring to the Code of Conduct (NMC, 2015) may be 5 minutes of your time each day at work. Factoring in time to record your evidence will be required. This should be as soon after the event as possible to aid your memory!

If I care about the people I care for, I have to do it

If nurses care about the people they nurse and want to serve them, then no matter what they have to do to revalidate, they will do it. Care and commitment (6Cs) relate to this. (Cummings, 2012)

People that are being cared for deserve to be nursed by registered nurses, and they can also provide feedback to the nurses. In fact, they do so in many ways every day. The challenge will be to capture this in a way that it can be viewed by the nurse as personal feedback to them and also incorporated into their portfolio and therefore their revalidation. Use the NMC feedback log forms. Points 2.3 and 3.3, plus the paragraph about patients and service users on page 3, (NMC, 2015) appear pertinent to the public.

In the 3 years, nurses must have a minimum of 5 pieces of feedback and to have reflected upon how this information has improved practice.

When people receive good care, in my experience, they are very pleased to acknowledge it and to thank the person who has provided it. They verbally say thank you; their non-verbal communication of a gesture, the way they look at you with gratitude; they write you a thank you note or card; they tell other staff how good they think that you are and without prompting. Mainly these are informal types of feedback.

Friends and family test; student evaluation; Care Quality Commission (CQC) results to the team; University research assessment exercise; hospital rating; are all means of feedback to teams. What other types of formal feedback has your team received?

Should nurses ask patients and/or their relatives/family/friends to provide feedback? Is it appropriate whilst they are still being nursed? Might they feel too scared to tell the truth in case it negatively impacts their care? How can they provide feedback and be anonymous, wouldn't that be open to nurses writing their own thank you notes? I have to ask, as nurses are human and as open to temptation as anyone else.

Gaining information from people you nurse is a formal requirement of revalidation and the NMC (2016a) provide information in Guidance Sheet 1. The Data Protection act is referred to as legal rules about storing people's data are covered by the Act, so the NMC advise that no names or other identifiable data is stored in your paper or electronic portfolio. It is recognised the confirmer's details will be in your portfolio and that is acceptable, since they have given consent.

It is unfortunate that no mention of how people could give their consent, for example to have a thank you note with their name on it included.

There is the issue of consent of other nurses having their names included, when documenting they have taken part in a participatory session or discussion. Also whether this falls under the Data Protection Act.

As revalidation is a slightly different process to the PREP process, it is inevitable that new information about how to achieve the process will emerge as nurses revalidate. Pilot sites were used and information extrapolated, but they involved small numbers of nurses and midwives, whereas the roll-out from April 2016 will obviously involve larger numbers.

For updates visit: www.NurseRevalidationBook.co.uk

Simple versus complicated

Who would refuse a KISS? Revalidation seems very complicated and a huge amount of extra work to some nurses. It can be simple - make it part of your practice and as little work as possible. Keeping It Simple Succeeds - the K.I.S.S. principle.

Life can be extremely complex and the aim of revalidation with ease is to keep things simple. Complicated makes things more difficult, simple makes things more easeful. Most of this chapter is about having a plan; setting intentions and keeping them; completing your intentions in the time you wanted to. That sounds simple, because it is meant to be.

Intentions are often called goals. Bradbury (2013) suggests using the word 'intentions' [or sometimes 'promises' instead] because they have a subtly different sound and feel to them. In fact, promising yourself something is linked to investing in yourself and can feel so much more achievable. Goals sound hard. Promising yourself something sounds more like giving yourself a gift and that can be so much easier to do. Additionally, if I promise to do something, I try extremely hard not to break that promise.

Whatever they are called, it is good to have a structure or process for them. The following acronym is one that many people have found helpful and you may have read about before.

S.M.A.R.T.
Specific (could also be Simple)
Measurable (Simple is often easier to measure)
Achievable (Simple is often easier to achieve)
Relevant (Simple is often more relevant)
Time-limited (Specific dates or time periods in which to succeed keeps the process Simple)
Ambler (2006) cited in Kerridge (2012).

Even though change is a feature of our lives every day, people often fear it or are resistant to it thinking that staying the same is somehow more comfortable. This seldom leads to growth (Kline, 2002). Resistance is often discussed with regard to changes others want you to undertake. For example, the NMC (2016a) changing the way that nurses retain their registration is others telling us what we need to do. (Kerridge, 2012). Although in fact, it builds on the PREP premise and is similar, just with clearer criteria and a structured framework. It can be that we introduce change and then resist our own changes! Being a resistor can complicate life, so it goes against the plan to use the K.I.S.S. principle and keep life simple. Go with the change, good things may happen when you step out of your 'comfort zone'! (Bradbury, 2013)

Getting support

This is about asking for help and receiving it (Bradbury, 2013) and mirrored in Point 13.3 (NMC, 2015)

This should be Simple (following on from previous points), however, it invariably is not! Some of this is linked to our feelings of self-worth and self-esteem, not to mention our self-confidence in asking for something for ourselves (Dickson, 2015). This may also be because asking for help can be interpreted as a sign of weakness, whereas acknowledging our ignorance should be recognised as a sign of strength. Team work is often espoused in the healthcare sector as the best way to benefit the people who we are caring for, therefore it makes sense to ask team members for help as no individual can know everything.

Time management. Put dates and times in your diary you will use for yourself to ensure that you progress in your career. You are the only person who can invest in you to meet the demands of your revalidation. Share your intentions timetable. When you have your intentions set with clear dates to meet them, others can help you be accountable for completion. Setting boundaries about how people assist you is a good idea, as the ideal would be they do it with love. When you accomplish your intention on, or before, the date you intended to you should request the people supporting you provide praise for your achievement. If you have been unable to complete your intention, then you need to request praise for any part of it that you have attained. Gentle probing to discover why you had difficulties succeeding and offers of help to meet a new date are the type of assistance that you will find most useful.

Peer support can be colleagues who you work with. Ask colleagues to cover your work whilst you undertake participatory study, or ask them to participate in study with you for mutual benefit. A reflective discussion partner is a suggested person to have (NMC, 2016a). It can be the same person as your confirmer (normally your line manager, if that person is a nurse) or a different person. It would seem sensible to have a separate reflective discussion partner and to pick someone with whom you meet easily, unless you have frequent and easy access to your confirmer.

Your confirmer can assist you in your accountability. Negotiate dates and times to meet with them as you travel on your revalidation journey, but you should initiate this and not expect them to. Involving them early in the process will enhance the relationship and enable them to see your progress. (RCN 2016)

Explain to friends in your immediate circle why occasionally you may have to see them slightly less often, whilst you concentrate on your learning and retaining your registration. Make it clear they are important to you and you value their friendship, also that you know they reciprocate.

Family. Ask them to only make reasonable demands on your time and to accept that you will require time for yourself. Share your 'timetable' with them, so they know when you are unavailable.

Ask all of the above to steer you back on course if you drift away from meeting the dates to complete your intentions. People who love and like you are usually pleased and flattered to be able to assist you, as it gives them a 'feel good' sensation. They may be waiting for you to ask for their help. Refusing their help may be hurtful to them, as they may feel you do not consider them good enough to help you. (Bradbury 2013)

Communication is key. Explain how important retaining your nurse registration is to you. Give simple, specific examples (see Chapter 2.5). Lastly, avoid sabotaging your own best efforts. This is when instead of spending time with, and on, yourself you allow the other things that need doing to distract you (Holt, 2012).

References:
Bradbury L (Ed) (2013) *The F Factor.* CreateSpace Independent Publishing Platform.
Baratta S (2014) *Simple Success. In business and in life.* Willow Tree 3.
Cummings J (2012) *Compassion in Practice. Nursing, midwifery and care staff. Our vision for the future.* London. Department of Health.
Dickson A (2015) *A woman in your own right: assertiveness and you.* London. Quartet Books.
Holt L (2012) *Get out of your own way. Stop sabotaging your business and learn to stand out in a crowded market.* London. National Alliance of Business Owners.
Kerridge J (2012) *Leading change: 2 – planning.* Nursing Times; 108 (5) Jan: 23-25.
Kline N (2002) *Time to think. Listening to ignite the human mind.* London. Cassell.
NMC (2015) *Revalidation. How to revalidate with the NMC. Requirements for renewing your registration.* London. NMC.
NMC (2016a) Revalidation. *How to revalidate with the NMC. Requirements for renewing your registration.* London. NMC.
Oakley A (1986) *Telling the truth about Jerusalem.* Oxford. Blackwell.

Claire Picton

Redgrave S & Townsend N (2005) *You can win at life! Unlock your potential and go for gold...* London. BBC Books.

www.NurseRevalidationBook.co.uk

Chapter 3
Planning your future career development

Study for career development

The word study sometimes seems like hard work and can be off-putting. The thing about life is we learn something new every day and we do not call it study. Your career development consists of informal and formal learning. The trick is to capture the informal learning and make it part of your revalidation, as that is the greater part of how learning in nursing occurs. The formal learning on courses and study days, by reading and completing online work or quizzes is useful too, but it then needs to be integrated into your daily practice.

The other aim is to make learning fun. Humour makes most things bearable in this life, so it is worth considering how studying can be joy-giving and fun-filled. It can be hard to do this alone, so shared learning is crucial. The participatory learning has to be shared, consider how it can also be enjoyable!

There also needs to be a clear focus on your learning and you have to believe that you are important enough to take time to learn. You also have to believe that it is within you to learn. If you are an under-confident person, then it may be that you need to develop the confidence to believe in yourself; so that you can learn with ease. "Speak nicely to yourself, because you are listening" is an unattributed quote from FaceBook. For example, don't call yourself 'stupid' if you don't know or understand something, you are merely ignorant and need to learn. 'Stupid' is a word that implies it is an unchangeable state and it is a label. As a nurse we should not be judging or labelling people, so it is best not to do that to ourselves either.

Exercise 3: write down the things you learnt yesterday. It may be related to work or it may be related to life experience. Jot notes down, no need to write in sentences. Fun element – use lots of different coloured pens or font colours so the page looks bright and exciting and interesting. Buzan & Buzan`s (1995) MindMap style works quite well when trying to capture thoughts.

Taking ideas that are in your head and writing them down is a great way to feel that you have made a start. In my experience it is easier to process and make sense of your ideas if you can visually see them. Hence writing, or even drawing, them.

Question: what do you need to learn in order to revalidate? Knowing what continuing professional development (CPD) you will need helps you to plan what to study.

Exercise 4. Spend 10 minutes writing down the things you think you currently need to learn in order to complete the process of revalidation.

Examples:
- I need to learn about the process of revalidation.
- I need to learn more about my current work specialism.
- I need to develop my reflective writing.

What do you want to do with your career? What is your plan? How will you know that you have achieved what you want to achieve? Move on to the next chapter to plan.

For updates visit: www.NurseRevalidationBook.co.uk

Planning your study time and your career

Planning your career and your study time to achieve learning is vital in order to achieve your promises or intentions for yourself.

No matter where you are in your career, you have chosen to continue practising as a nurse or you would not be reading this book about revalidation. Unless you are reading it to assist other nurses to revalidate. Either way, the aim of this chapter is to make you think about your career and plan how you want it to develop.

Claire Picton

Why did you choose to become a nurse? Revisit exercise 2 in Chapter 1. What does the best nurse you could possibly be look like to you? How would you envisage yourself to be? How would others view you?

Action plan example:

Example Action plan:	To be achieved:	Ways to achieve:
Revalidation date [it will be on the first day of the month in which it is due].	Due 01/02/2017 Expires 28/02/2017	Complete online in the 60-day period [01/12/16 to 01/02/2017]
CPD Participatory Learning	20 hours	Monthly sessions planned with a group of the nurses where I work – alternating case study with journal article. Lecturing – interactive group work with nurses who are students [Associate Lecturer role]. Attending study days: Booked a 1-day conference (also presenting an interactive workshop) and attending RCN Congress 2016. Will be completed June 2016.
CPD Non-Participatory Learning	15 hours	Reading journal articles. Undertaking online quizzes.
Practice hours [only need planning if you are working part-time]	450 hours I work 22.5 hours per week. Need to work: 60 days – 20 weeks.	I will have no issues meeting this amount of hours. [Unless I have a long period of sick leave, in the future.]
Reflective Discussion Partner	Decided it will be my line manager, as I am a senior nurse in the organisation and it is more appropriate. I do have external peers who I can also undertake reflective discussion with.	Plan 20 minutes per week to discuss reflections on action.
Confirmer	Line manager.	
Reflective pieces	5	From clinical practice.

Table 5

Exercise 5. Make your own action plan and insert relevant dates for yourself. Share with your confirmer and your reflective discussion partner if you have both.

If you are a confirmer and/or a reflective discussion partner, ask to see the action plan of the nurse(s) who you are to confirm/partner in order for you to plan dates for your diary too. (Tomlinson, 2015)

What will you achieve from booking onto a course/study day?

Will booking onto a course or study day (programme) be a good investment for you? Not only of your time but of your money or your employers' money? Be discerning, write down any objectives that might be achieved from attending the programme. Contemplate how it will progress your Continuing Professional Development (CPD) in the long-term.

Discuss this with others if necessary, for example, your line manager or your reflective discussion partner.

The form below gives you some aspects that you need to think about.

	Considerations:	Actions:
Find a study day or course advertisement.	How appropriate is it for the area in which you are working? How is it going to improve or impact your practice? Is there a clear breakdown of the things that will be in the programme? What do you expect to get out of it? Do the objectives that they have match the objectives that you want to get out of the course? How far away is the venue? What time does it start and finish?	Decide whether to book it. This may involve a discussion with your employer.
	What's the time investment? [Including travelling time both ways, potential loss of day off.]	Ask employer if you can take study leave and have the actual day(s) away from work
	What is the financial investment? [Including transport, food and any accommodation costs, potential loss of earnings.]	Ask employer if they are willing to pay the whole cost; something, nothing.
If you decide to book.	Is the best investment in your time taking the train/coach so you can combine travel and work/relaxing? Is First Class travel the best investment if you are working whilst travelling?	Book travel that is suitable for working in or relaxing in. Book travel early to get cheaper tickets. Book accommodation PRN or stay with family/friends.
Attending	There will be networking opportunities with other attendees and with speakers.	Take objectives with you. Speak to people. Make notes. Reflect on the activity.
On return	Find time in diary to give feedback session. Provide an A4 summary for staff who cannot attend feedback session.	Put notes into portfolio. Prepare a feedback session for staff. Give feedback to staff – written and/or verbal.

Form 1

It may also be useful to put costings into the diagram, both of time and money.

Participatory Study Hours

The participatory study hours which make up 20 hours of continuing professional development (CPD) have to be completed over 3 years. The NMC does not prescribe how these will be achieved, but leaves it up to the individual practitioners. It will either consist of courses, study days, or potentially things that you do in practice. Practice may be clinical, managerial or educational and you must consider the types of things that are most relevant to you. Relevant points 6.1; 6.2; 13.5; 19.2; 22.3 (NMC, 2015)

Think about activities you can undertake with other nurses you could use as participatory time and how you capture that detail. The form below could be used and signed by all the staff who participated – providing they give written consent. Otherwise, simply add the number of staff and whether they were nurses, doctors or allied health professionals; they may wish to have a copy for their portfolio.

Participatory Study			
Date:		
Topic discussed:		
Summary of discussion:		
Implications for practice:		
References:		
Time taken:		
Only use this, with names, if it does not contravene the Data Protection Act (1998) I consent to this being inserted into the portfolio of each contributor:			
Staff signature. Print Name.	Staff signature. Print Name.	Staff signature. Print Name.
Staff signature. Print Name.	Staff signature. Print Name.	Staff signature. Print Name.
		Form 2

If at handover you have some brief teaching or discussion about the management of a particular person's care, that may count. It is important to capture the time, however short, since 20 hours over three years is a short period of time. It equates to 400 minutes (6 hours 40 minutes) per year, so 10 minutes of participatory discussion at 40 handovers would provide you with sufficient time. Although it is probably better to have a mixture of learning.

Case conferences or ward rounds about patients, for example; informal discussion of patient care between two or more Healthcare Professionals (HCPs); a student's progress or managing staff count as participatory study; as would a journal club; teaching sessions, either formal or informal; reflective discussions; if you are mentoring a student participatory discussion will occur and you can learn from the student as well; curriculum planning; planning service improvements. Again it is about thinking creatively about how you capture that time and record it as evidence.

There are lots of participatory hours that probably occur during the day and the challenge is to be able to document them as evidence for your portfolio. It is therefore about recognising when they occur then making the effort and taking the time to document. This may be writing a very brief paragraph or two relating to what you have talked about with colleagues. Remember to mention references and/or what evidence you have used.

It is important to have a range of people that you discuss with, as you would not just talk with student nurses or nurses who are your peers since that might limit your learning. Discussions with members of the multidisciplinary team (MDT) and more senior nurses, perhaps nurse educators from the University would probably help you demonstrate wider, and perhaps deeper, learning. To have variety and a different way of learning from each other makes it more interesting and less repetitive.

The Continuing Professional Development (CPD) Log template form can be found on the revalidation micro-site of the NMC, the link is at: www.NurseRevalidationBook.co.uk

Non-participatory Study Hours

The non-participatory study hours comprise 15 hours of CPD in 3 years. Individual practitioners can choose how to accomplish these. Non participatory hours for CPD are solitary study, remember to note how long they took you to complete each time you finish them. The table on page 42 gives some examples.

Examples are:	Action [including time taken to complete it]:
Reflection	Only 5 reflections have to be discussed, others can be written. Insert in portfolio, ensuring entries are anonymous.
Reading	Write a summary of what you read, how useful it will be to your practice and note the full reference. Insert in portfolio. Share the written summary with other staff for them to read. This might help them know whether the book or article contained useful information and whether in your opinion it would make a difference to future practice.
Online quiz	Complete and put into portfolio. Note URL to share with other staff.
Questionnaires	Complete and put into portfolio.
Teaching programmes and/or E-learning packages.	Use and work through on your own. Your organisation may have produced their own. External companies may have produced them. Devise a teaching package for others, designed to be used in a non-participatory manner. Insert into portfolio.
CPD articles with questions	Complete and send to journal (if it is an option). Obtain answers from a subsequent edition of the Journal. Insert into portfolio.
Write a letter to a journal about an article you have read.	Copy the page from the Journal that it is published in and insert in portfolio.
Write an article, as you have to read the literature to do so.	Copy the published article and insert in portfolio.
Write a report that requires a literature search.	Minutes of meeting where your report is presented, inserted in portfolio. Anonymous entries if necessary.
Writing a lesson plan.	Devise a lesson plan and include a copy in your portfolio.
Write a book	Letter from publisher congratulating you on publication inserted in your portfolio.
Simulation teaching.	This may have a lesson plan. There may be photographs and/or video. Electronic storage can hold these.
Making informational videos.	Video. Electronic storage can hold these.
Devising scenarios &/or OSCEs.	Copy the scenarios and insert in portfolio.

Table 6

Relevant points 6.1; 6.2; 13.5; 19.2; 22.3 (NMC, 2015)

Forms to capture this data are available on the website: www.NurseRevalidationBook.co.uk

Evaluating the benefits of your study

All the exercises in this book so far have shown you how to evaluate what you have learnt, so this is just an overview of thinking about how you might capture in one place the continuing professional development you have successfully undertaken.

Below is a form that allows you to document your continuing professional development concisely. It also enables you to cross-reference within your portfolio exactly where your different types of evidence are stored, because when you come to look at your portfolio with your confirmer it will make life easier (Chapter 2). Also when you're reviewing your portfolio or you want to share your study with other people, it makes it simpler to navigate through your portfolio.

The main thing to remember is that you are not studying just to go through the process of revalidation (NMC, 2016a), the point is for you to progress and develop because it is your continuing professional development. It will enable you to review and look at your CPD and look at the huge amount you have achieved over the last three years.

It can be useful then for you to take to an interview. A one-page sheet giving the information about the sort of study you have undertaken shows that you have planned for your personal development review and/or job interview. It highlights that you take your continuing professional development extremely seriously and that you want to share it with other people as well. Never underestimate how important your learning is but how important flagging up your learning to other people you work with is too, it is a very powerful tool to demonstrate just how committed and what an excellent nurse you are because you're learning all the time. So well done you! It is also a powerful motivator to do even more learning as you can see how confident and successful it makes you.

Type of evidence:	Dates updated/completed:	Filed in portfolio section:
Curriculum Vitae	Updated on	Personal Details
Record of participatory study hours (use NMC form)	Completed on	CPD - participatory
Record of non-participatory study hours (use NMC form)	Completed on	CPD - non-participatory
Reflective pieces (use NMC form)	Completed on	Reflections
Feedback (use NMC form)	Completed on	Feedback
Discussions with RDP/confirmer (use NMC form)	Completed on	Reflective Discussions

Table 7

References:

Buzan T & Buzan B (1995) *The Mind Map Book.* London. BBC Books.

NMC (2015) Code of Conduct. London. NMC.

NMC (2016a) *Revalidation. How to revalidate with the NMC. Requirements for renewing your registration.* London. NMC.

Rogers C & Freiberg HJ (1994) *Freedom to learn.* 3rd Ed. London. Prentice Hall.

Tomlinson C (2015) *Revalidation for Nurses and Midwives. A Handbook for Registrants.* U.K. Amazon.

www.NurseRevalidationBook.co.uk

Chapter 4
Daily work and revalidation

Give us this day – exploiting opportunities at work

Each day finding opportunities at work and then exploit them for your learning. Both for participatory and non-participatory study Continuing Professional Development (CPD).

As a nurse you have to be healthy enough to perform your role - point 20.9 (NMC, 2015) For ease, look after yourself and undertake self-care daily. This is not only ensuring good nutrition, hydration and exercise for physical fitness, but attending to your psychosocial wellbeing too (Richardson, 2009, Pegram & Bloomfield, 2015).

If you work part-time, then you must record your hours to ensure you undertake 450 hours over 3 years. Full-time nurses will accrue sufficient hours. These relate to point 22.2 (NMC, 2015).

Weave learning into your working day. How can you do this? Daily practice is rich in evidence and will provide you with incidents you can reflect on.

What is understood by clinical practice? Not all nurses work directly with patients. Managers and educationalists are more likely to indirectly affect patient care by imparting their knowledge and expertise to the staff who do directly work with patients. Indirect care is still part of nursing, if you are required to hold current registration in order to manage or educate, there is not a requirement for managers and educators to obtain 450 direct clinical practice hours simply work hours. It is always an advantage to spend some time in clinical practice, even if that is in a supervisory capacity, to experience something of the nature of clinical work now – it may have changed out of recognition since you were giving direct care. Managers are particularly likely to be confirmers, so it can help to provide a realistic view of the pressures the nurse you are confirming is experiencing.

NMC Code of Conduct (2015) has to be a theme throughout your revalidation process. Therefore, you need to become familiar with it. Display it, or have it easily accessible in your workplace and refer to it often. Point 20.1 NMC (2015)

The Code is divided into 4 sections – see page 47. It is separated further into 25 points, which in turn are sub-divided. Please refer to the full Code of Conduct (NMC, 2015).

NMC Code of Conduct (2015)
Prioritise people.
• You put the interests of people using or needing nursing or midwifery services first. • You make their care and safety your main concern and make sure that their dignity is preserved and their needs are recognised, assessed and responded to. • You make sure that those receiving care are treated with respect, that their rights are upheld and that any discriminatory attitudes and behaviours towards those receiving care are challenged.
Practise effectively.
~ You assess need and deliver or advise on treatment, or give help [including preventative or rehabilitative care] without too much delay and to the best of your abilities, on the basis of the best evidence available and best practice. ~ You communicate effectively, keeping clear and accurate records and sharing skills, knowledge and experience where appropriate. ~ You reflect and act on any feedback you receive to improve your practice.
Preserve safety.
o You make sure that patient and public safety is protected. o You work within the limits of your competence, exercising your professional 'duty of candor' and raising concerns immediately whenever you come across situations that put patients or public safety at risk. o You take necessary action to deal with any concerns where appropriate.
Promote professionalism and trust.
• You uphold the reputation of your profession at all times. • You should display a personal commitment to the standards of practice and behaviour set out in the code. • You should be a model of integrity and leadership for others to aspire to. This should lead to trust and confidence in the profession from patients, people receiving care, other healthcare professionals and the public.
NMC (2015)

Gaining evidence for revalidation from your workplace

Reflection is the most obvious form of evidence, but there are other ways and they probably involve peers, colleagues, managers, other Health Care Professionals (HCPs) giving you written feedback. This can be concise and need not be a lengthy process for the other HCPs.

Suggestions from NMC (2016b) include:
- Clinical supervision documents
- Clinical audit participation – a letter stating how you were involved
- Clinical research; minutes of meetings (anonymous entries)
- Clinical practice visits to areas other than your normal clinical practice
- Job training opportunities, including - shadowing of other HCPs, rotation and/or secondment
- Written letters from other HCPs
- Coaching – being coached or coaching others.
- Mentoring – being mentored or mentoring others.

In addition:
- Active participation in handover.
- Developing information leaflets for patients and their families.
- Developing and producing orientation packages for student nurses who come to your clinical area on placement.
- Developing and creating orientation packages for new staff.
- Developing and creating learning packages for staff in your clinical area.
- Researching a subject and giving a teaching session or presentation to other staff about it.
- Care Quality Commission feedback report.
- Minutes of meetings you attend that relate to the functioning of the organisation/business in which you undertake your work.

- Writing reports. The whole report does not need to be included, but evidence that you were a contributor would suffice.
- Teaching on a course in a University.
- Curriculum development, usually in a University.
- Writing and giving a presentation, within your organisation.
- Being short-listed for a workplace award.
- Being a judge for a workplace award.

Evidence from any of the above will go into your portfolio.

An example from clinical practice for nurses giving direct care is reporting deterioration in patients. It is useful to think in a logical sequence and the **A**irway **B**reathing **C**irculation **D**isability **E**xposure [ABCDE] format is a good one to use in clinical practice (Resuscitation Council, 2011). Use specific language that other Healthcare Professionals (HCPs) can understand, rather than vague terms. For example, 'although this patient's observations are within normal parameters at the moment, the history and my visual observations of the patient indicate to me that they are compensating but in, or about to go into, a peri-arrest state and need immediate treatment' would be a better statement of the situation than 'the patient looks very unwell and I'm worried about them'. (Smith et al, 2011)

There are useful tools for meaningful and safe handover and the following are two examples:

1. SBAR **S**ituation, **B**ackground, **A**ssessment, **R**ecommendation [SBAR] (Resuscitation Council (UK), 2011).
2. RSVP **R**eason, **S**tory, **V**ital Signs, **P**lan [RSVP] (Resuscitation Council (UK), 2011).

Participatory activities could include handover, as it is where discussion and teaching may well occur. A case conference about a patient, and this may include their relatives, is another example of a participatory activity. Discussion about a student nurse and their progress might be an educator's participatory activity. Managers may discuss complaints or project management as their participatory activity. It is important to record how long the participatory activity takes. Guidance Sheet 3 (NMC, 2016b) gives examples and information about what is a Continuing Professional Development (CPD) activity.

Discussions with your confirmer will assist both of you to understand what is a possible, achievable and sensible CPD activity that occurs in your area of clinical practice. A wider dialogue with other nurses in that same area may reveal ideas and information you and your confirmer had not considered.

The art of nursing

Art – use your creative side to imagine ways of gaining evidence of your participatory Continuing Professional Development (CPD) throughout your clinical practice and work.

Nurses are highly creative, they take what seems like impossible situations in their daily clinical practice and turn them into positive and safe outcomes for the staff and patients they work with every day. Practising effectively often means using creative communication and one's imagination, particularly when caring for people who are distressed or cognitively impaired in some way.

If English is not the person's first language, then the nurse has to use language creatively, picking the words and or phrases that might be best understood and also using non-verbal communication including drawing and gesturing with hands or pointing to things to get the message across. Knowing when and where to obtain people who may be able to translate, which may occasionally be relatives but are more likely to be staff who understand medical terms in their native language or formal interpreters [Points 7.2, 7.3 & 7.4 (NMC, 2015)].

Bringing love and light to every situation is creative (Bradbury, 2013). Sometimes it is difficult to do if the patient is dying or has a poor prognosis, but it can be extremely rewarding to assist someone to have a good death and to be able to creatively support the relatives as well. I have seen nurses create a home-like environment in a side-room, when a patient was unable to fulfil their wishes to go home to die.

Dealing with a student who is failing to achieve and has left it until very close to their assignment submission date to seek assistance. Lecturers may have to give feedback that limits the amount of revisions so that they can be achieved in the time-scale available. This may mean the student is only likely to attain the minimum mark to pass the course work, but it is the realistic result that can be created in the circumstances. Presenting this solution with love and light needs to be crafted skilfully, particularly if the student has unrealistic expectations of obtaining 80% or more!

Managers spend the majority of their work being creative around staffing and working to provide the best staffing levels possible given the various demands; staff needing time for statutory and mandatory training, staff having to take time off for annual leave, sick leave, emergency care leave, bereavement leave, leave for jury service and maternity/paternity leave. The financial constraints they work with means there has to be a huge amount of creative thinking when managing budgets and staffing, not to mention other resources.

Exercise 6. Write down the creative aspects you have incorporated into your work recently and how it has improved practice. This probably links best with Practising effectively (NMC, 2015)

Buddying up in your daily work

Know who your supporters and encouragers are at work and use them as much as possible, ask for help and receive it from them. Team work allows mutual support. Use your confirmer and your Reflective Discussion Partner as well. There is a need for trust here, which can be difficult for some people to do, especially letting go of control and trusting others (Bradbury, 2013).

Make a list of the people who you would ask for support and write beside their name the specific type of assistance you think you require or would be able to get from them. If they are nurses this could be reciprocal evidence for your mutual portfolios, although they do not have to be nurses.

Examples are given in Table 8.

Name of staff member who can support me:	Specific support they might give:	Agreed: Yes or No
Line Manager.	To be Confirmer for my revalidation. To be my reflective discussion partner (RDP) [optional]. To meet monthly for me to show examples from my portfolio; for me to state any goals, promises, intentions I have made for myself to achieve in the forthcoming month. To help me keep accountable for my actions.	Yes
Peer.	To share articles, professional websites that we might find mutually beneficial for our revalidation and CPD. Possibly share what we have learnt from our reading and have participatory discussions about aspects of your clinical practice. To be my reflective discussion partner (RDP) [optional].	
Nurse who is undertaking the same course as you.	As for peer, but also you can both discuss the assignment(s) and course work that you need to complete in order to successfully pass your course.	
Colleague who is junior.	Support by agreeing to be mentored or coached by you.	
Colleague who is senior.	Clinical supervision.	
A non-nurse HCP.	Knowledge about others in the Multi-Disciplinary Team who also care for the same patients you do. For example: paramedics; doctors; Speech and Language therapists; radiographers; business managers. Or perhaps teach the same student nurses. For example: biologists; pharmacists; simulation specialists; moulage specialists.	

Table 8

The list in Table 8 is not exhaustive and only you will be able to create your own list. It is simply to help if you are having difficulty getting started – so you may not even need it!

Once you have made the list, it is useful to have a brief meeting or conversation with each person so that they know the following:

- You need support.
- You think they are the person who can give you support.
- They have the opportunity to accept or decline your request.

The pair of you may have to do some work to consider how, what, where, and when that support will be given and the format it will take. Written agreements are usually best to help keep you on track and accountable [see also Chapter 2].

People generally like to be asked to help, especially if they are nurses. Helping is what nurses do, after all. Where there is a need to ask for help, it is likely that some nurses have to learn to receive that help when it is offered/given (Bradbury, 2013). It also can give a feel-good factor to the person you are asking. Should the person be unable to support you due to other commitments, avoid taking it personally.

Team working

If there are differences in approaches, it is important to recognise them and seek ways to work together as a team. Team work is vital when dealing with patients seeking unscheduled care. There is nothing wrong with admitting the facts presented by the patient are not ones you are familiar with and that a discussion with a colleague might lead to a more accurate diagnosis, or the most appropriate way to treat the patient. Not knowing the answer is not failure, but failure to seek help can result in permanent harm to a patient. Point 13.2 (NMC, 2015). It also links with asking for help and receiving it (Bradbury, 2013).

Encourage yourself and others, do not judge (Bradbury, 2013)

Working with people is always challenging and they can be highly unpredictable. In order to make sense of our world, we often judge and stereotype to reduce some of the unpredictability. However, people then seldom behave according to the stereotype that we have assigned them, they therefore seem unpredictable. This is all getting much too complicated, so why not go back to the Keep It Simple Successfully (K.I.S.S.) principle? [see Chapter 2.]

Praise more than you criticise. When you criticise make it constructive criticism that can be learnt from and action taken to improve the situation either now or in the future. Encourage people to learn something every day, including something about themselves (Richardson, 2009)

Encouraging people feels good. It usually makes them smile and be happy and pleased. When people smile, it is infectious and makes others smile too. Smiling makes people feel good. Encourage people to follow their dreams (Colvin, 2008).

Exercise 7. What are your dreams? What is your passion? If you know what these are it is easier to ascertain what your purpose in life is and to journey towards achieving it.

When you are praised, say thank you and smile, be grateful. Avoid putting yourself down, because that is also like refusing the praise. That may make the other person feel their praise was rejected, that they have been rejected, they feel unhappy because they were trying to help and that help was perceived negatively.

Encourage people to undertake a risk assessment of their fears (Baratta, 2014).

Exercise 8. What are your fears? How do they distract you from journeying towards your purpose?

The reflective discussion partner and the confirmer should cultivate their mentoring and coaching skills, especially in encouraging staff (Elock & Sharples, 2011). Points: 6.2; 9.1; 9.3; 20.8 (NMC, 2015).

Exercise 9. Think back and make a note of the times you have encouraged people at work and the ways you have done it. Contemplate whether it has been effective. If possible, ask the people if they found the encouragement useful and if so – how. If it was unhelpful, ask them to explain why in order to allow you to learn.

The science of nursing

We mentioned having a purpose in chapter 4. The science of nursing relates to being logical, planning ahead, being pro-active, measuring your progress. [see Chapter 3] devising action plans and SMART objectives [see Chapter 2]. All of these can assist you in keeping yourself accountable for your actions.

This is about using objective measures in order to work out what is being done, then to use logic. In relation to clinical nursing, it would be taking observations that you can measure; respiratory rate, heart rate, blood pressure, and temperature. These are recordable and measurable and you can compare with subsequent readings that you take. And they can also be subjective and you can apply some objective measures, the most common one being a pain rating scale (analogue), when you have an initial measurement for that person you can then compare the person's subsequent scores to their initial score. You cannot extrapolate it then use the score to compare with other people's, for example, my pain rating score of 10 will not equal anyone else's pain rating score of 10, they are not comparable. However, if I say my pain rating scale is 10 then I am given analgesia and 30 minutes later I am asked my pain rating score again, this time I say it is 8, obviously the analgesia has had some effect. Therefore, it is measurable against the benchmark at the beginning. Your progress can be actual things then or it could also be measuring yourself against the first benchmark that you set out.

Measuring your progress might be important and one way to do that is to develop action plans and then have cut-off dates for completing tasks. That helps you keep yourself accountable for your actions, one of the things about being responsible for yourself is actually making sure you are responsible for your own learning and that is quite a broad topic. Breaking it down into an action plan, for example: I want to go on the study day; I want to evaluate whether it's worth me doing it by a specific date; then if I decide it is worth doing I will book it by a specific date; I will attend it on the date of the study day and then I will evaluate whether the study day was useful and whether there are things I can take back to my workplace by a specific date after the study day, preferably within one or two days of the study day. Capturing that sort of information soon after the study day means you will be less likely to forget things. It would be helpful during this study day or immediately afterwards to make brief notes about what you are going to present as feedback to other people in your workplace. Also using SMART objectives, see chapter 2, for measuring your progress see chapter 3.

Exercise 10. In what ways do you use science in your work and how does it help you? Make notes and reflect.

References

Baratta S (2014) *Simple Success. In business and in life.* Willow Tree 3.

Bradbury L (Ed) (2013) *The F Factor.* CreateSpace Independent Publishing Platform.

Colvin G (2008) *Talent is overrated: what really separates world-class performers from everyone else.* Nicholas Brealey Publishing Ltd.

Elock K and Sharples K (2011) *A Nurses Survival Guide to Mentoring* London. Churchill Livingston Elsevier.

NMC (2015) *Code of Conduct.* London. NMC.

NMC (2016b) *How to revalidate booklet. Guidance Sheet 3 Examples of CPD activities.* NMC. London.

Pegram A & Bloomfield J (2015) *Nutrition and fluid management* Nursing Standard 29(31) 1-7 Apr: 38-42.

Resuscitation Council (UK) (2011) *Advanced Life Support 6th Ed.* London. Resuscitation Council (UK)

Richardson C (2009) *The art of extreme self-care: transform your life one month at a time.* London. Hay House.

Rogers C & Freiberg HJ (1994) *Freedom to learn. 3rd Ed.* London. Prentice Hall.

Smith S, Adam D. Kirkpatrick P & McRobie (2011) *Using solution-focused communication to support patients* Nursing Standard 31 Aug:42-47

www.NurseRevalidationBook.co.uk

Chapter 5
Will the registered nurse step up and shine please?

Embrace your imperfections and learn from them

Can you do this? Yes, you can.

Exercise 11: Take a sheet of A4 paper and fold it in half. Write on one half 'Strengths' and on the other half 'Areas for development'. In my experience, many people write strengths and weaknesses. The reason I use the term 'Areas for development' is because I have found that people have negative emotional responses to the word 'weaknesses'. If you are to succeed it is best to react positively to it.

The first thing to write under strengths is the most positive thing for your revalidation – that is:

Registered Nurse

Now that has got you started, please continue, but try and alternate writing strengths and areas for development. This is to try and avoid one side of the page having loads more on it than the other side.

When you have finished, read your strengths out loud. Congratulate yourself on having all those strengths! You are amazing! Believe you are the credible and effective registered nurse that you are.

It is human to make mistakes and the risk assessment is to reduce, not eliminate, the likelihood of mistakes being made.

In my experience, most nurses strive to achieve Gold standard (or ideal/best possible) care for all the patients they encounter in their clinical practice. It is worth guarding against believing that all patients have to receive gold standard care regardless of the context in which they are receiving that care. Within healthcare services, it is unlikely that all the conditions for providing optimal care will always be present. Nurses need to recognise this and to therefore understand that sometimes they can only provide safe care, or somewhere between safe care and gold standard care. Safe care is always acceptable and it is good. For example, if there is an unusually high volume of patients requiring care and staffing is sub-optimal due to sickness, annual leave, maternity leave, special leave and/or absence then it is perfectly acceptable to be giving safe care. Sometimes the staff working do not possess all the skills required to provide gold standard care. Nurses should not berate themselves for this, but recognise that it is a necessity. Perfection is something to aim for, but it is not a necessity. Mostly care given is somewhere between safe and Gold standard (diagram 1) and that is fine.

If care becomes unsafe that is a different issue entirely and needs escalation to senior staff, verbally initially and then usually followed up in writing. This relates to the preserving safety section of the NMC (2015) Code of Conduct. Many UK NHS Trusts have the electronic system DATIX for incident reporting, but all organisations will have some mechanisms for reporting incidents and it is your responsibility to know what you have to use in your workplace. To be proactive, escalation may be necessary when care is hovering around the border between safe and unsafe.

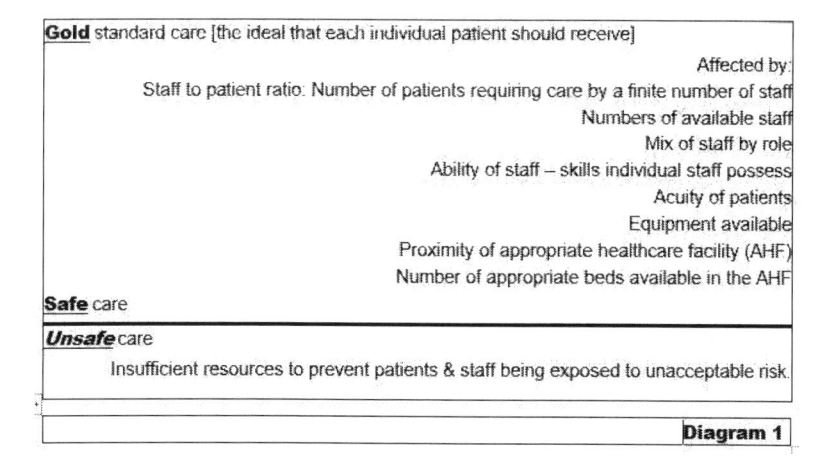

Gold standard care [the ideal that each individual patient should receive]
Affected by:
Staff to patient ratio: Number of patients requiring care by a finite number of staff
Numbers of available staff
Mix of staff by role
Ability of staff – skills individual staff possess
Acuity of patients
Equipment available
Proximity of appropriate healthcare facility (AHF)
Number of appropriate beds available in the AHF
Safe care
Unsafe care
Insufficient resources to prevent patients & staff being exposed to unacceptable risk.
Diagram 1

This is important because having unachievable expectations can lead to disillusionment and unnecessary stress (Wicks, 2005).

Exercise 12. Write down what realistic expectations have you had at work this week.

What works for you, as the RN stepping up and shining?

When you go to work, walk in with your head held high and look confident and as though you mean to be there. You may wonder what this has to do with revalidation, but if you are to succeed with your revalidation you have to believe that you are successful and can remain on the register.

Self-care is a vital part of your daily ritual and should not be an optional extra when you have served everyone else (Richardson, 2009, Bradbury, 2013). Planning in your diary to undertake 2-4 of these each day allows you to increase your self-worth and confidence.

Self-care examples	
Read Bible and bible notes and spend time with God and in prayer.	Spend time in a Spa.
Have a foot-spa at home [in dining room or on decking in nice weather!]	Use the steam shower room.
Relax in the hot tub.	Listen to music.
Go out into the outdoors/nature. Appreciate creation.	Walk.
15 minutes on stationary bike or rowing machine.	15 minutes rebounding.
Dance whilst listening to music.	Swim or water jog.
Read a book.	Write in my journal.
Contact a family member or a friend: write a letter; send a text; use WhatsApp; use FaceBook; ring them up.	
Have hair done.	Have a pedicure.
	Table 9

Exercise 13. List the things that are important in your self-care. They are best if they are things that fill you with deep joy.

The people you work with and interact with expect you to be confident in your role, although that should never preclude you from asking for help – point 13.3 (NMC, 2015); to be kind to each other, that is what we are paid for in the NHS; to keep yourself safe – point 13.4 (NMC, 2015).

If you are having a bad day, then pick someone who you can confide in. This may be a colleague, your line manager, or someone from the chaplaincy team or occupational health team. Work out how you can deal with your problems without them impacting on those you work with and remain at work.

The confirmer needs to have the skills to encourage and ideally should have a relationship with the nurse who they are acting as confirmer for. Otherwise you will only have 60 days before the registered nurse's revalidation date to meet up and to confirm that the RGN has successfully undertaken the process of revalidation.

Be organised and have the evidence for your revalidation ready in good time.

Don't expect to be perfect, but do expect to shine despite your imperfections. It may not be every minute of every day, although certainly at some points every day.

Filling yourself up first, personally and professionally

What do you do that makes you feel like the most effective, caring, compassionate, professional nurse possible?

Exercise 14. Write down the things you do when you are preparing to go to work and then also when you arrive in the workplace that makes you feel like the nurse you want to be? Some nurses like to arrive early so they can mentally prepare, by 'switching off' from their personal life and getting into their nurse role/persona. Some have rituals they undertake on arrival. One useful ritual is to either mentally map out or write down what you aim to achieve that day at work. As you are thinking about revalidation, add in how you might achieve one aspect of the revalidation process.

Simply by attending work you are automatically adding hours worked towards your goal of 450 hours over 3 years. Is there anything in your work day that would contribute time towards your 20 hours of participatory learning/study? Is there time out that you take in your work day to undertake any of the individual learning that would form part of your 15 hours of non-participatory study?

Your body is where you live and meeting its physical needs are paramount. Nutrition and hydration are as vital for staff, as for the clientele they care for. Yet how often do we hear nurses say they have not had time for a break? That they just grab 'food on the go' (Pegram & Bloomfield, 2015). Ensuring you plan and take the breaks you are entitled to is important, both physically and mentally. Maintaining your own health is a requirement to practice as a nurse, point 20.9 (NMC, 2015). In order to take them you will probably have to ask for help and trust that other nurses, or staff, can cover for you (Bradbury, 2013).

Looking for positives in your daily work

Exercise 15. At the end of your work day, think of at least three positive things that have happened, or three things where you know you have made a difference to a patient, a relative, another nurse, a co-worker, another member of the multidisciplinary team (MDT). Make a habit of doing this daily.

End of work time positive aspects capture form.	
During this time at work I have:	Examples:
Clinical example 1)	Looked after Mrs X and she thanked me for taking the time to ensured her hair was washed and brushed into a nice style before her husband came to visit.
Clinical example 2)	The medical registrar thanked me for contacting her/him pro-actively to highlight the deterioration in Mr Y's physical condition [using National Early Warning System (NEWS)] and enabling early treatment aimed at improving Mr Y's condition.
Clinical example 3)	I was able to explain to other staff about something they did not know and they were pleased to have received the information and teaching.
Manager example	Received a thank you letter from a relative about how the team on a ward, you have managerial responsibility for, provided great care. Senior manager in the organisation gave praise for a report produced.
Educator example	External examiner gives positive feedback on the quality of the assignments they have moderated. Student evaluations are positive about the course/module they have attended.

Form 3

The above can also help gain perspective and achieve balance on a difficult day when nothing seemed to have gone well, until you searched for and remembered the positives that did happen – no matter how small (Redgrave & Townsend, 2005).

Can any of these people write something for you to capture it? For example, the feedback from acting up into a different role under supervision. Or you can document feedback that you have received yourself.

Or it could be team feedback; a thank you card or note that is left for the team, positive feedback from a Care Quality Commission inspection, a team receiving an internal organisational or external award, positive feedback following a curriculum revalidation or a University research assessment exercise.

Always Events (Institute for Healthcare Improvement) "Always Events are aspects of the patient experience that are so important to patients and families that health care providers must perform them consistently for every patient, every time." This is focussing on positives in clinical practice, as opposed to the 'never events' that used to be concentrated on.

For updates visit: www.NurseRevalidationBook.co.uk

Being visible in your workplace

So what is it about being a registered nurse that marks you out as being different at work? From other types of staff, health care assistants? Or educators or managers, who are not nurses, depending obviously on your work setting. This goes back to what you were thinking about at the beginning of the book about what it means to be a nurse and what it means to you to be a nurse (see chapter 1). But it is about stepping up and shining even if you're not feeling great that day or you're not feeling like you're doing the best job, but recognising there are positive things you show and vibes you give off. Some of the confidence might be about your knowledge base, which leads back obviously to Continuing Practice Development (CPD) and therefore to revalidation and that is what we are talking about here! The more you know and are able to understand what you need to do at work then the more confident you are going to be and you will shine! You will show up as the most confident registered nurse whenever you work, in whatever role you are actually undertaking.

That does not mean that it is not ok for you to ask for help, because clearly it is always best to ask for help if you need it and is a sign of strength (Bradbury, 2013). Simply because you have successfully completed a lot of study or have been a registered nurse in your area of expertise for a long period of time does not mean that you need to know everything. I have spent 40 years as a nurse and I still do not know everything and I do not expect to know everything. Nobody can know everything. I do know who are the most appropriate people to ask for assistance.

The whole value of team work is asking other people and then accepting their help and going with what they say, except of course if you know they are actually wrong or about to put someone else in jeopardy. You have to be sure that it will not be detrimental to patient care, if you work in clinical practice.

Being a nurse might be about what being a nurse means to you as an individual. It might also be about the common characteristics of being a nurse and what this society understands about these. This relates back to the NMC (2015) Code of Conduct and how we show that we are practising effectively. Those are things in the paragraphs above in terms of knowledge - knowing and understanding what it is you are supposed to be doing at work. Then demonstrating that to others.

It is also related to making sure your confirmer knows who you are. You are being visible at work and you are not hiding your skills and expertise, so that they are able to see them and appreciate the good work you are undertaking. Showing up at work and making a difference in what you do. It might be the small things that make an impact, but it is that other people know you are at work and recognise that you have shown up and you are seen to be good at doing your job. You ask questions, you help people, and you serve them as well as serving yourself.

What is different about a confirmer?

Being visible as a nurse is likely to also attract positive feedback about you (and your team), which is what you require to revalidate. A confirmer is likely to be a confident leader who is respectful of their team members (Kline, 2002).

Being a role model

Exercise 16. Write notes about what being a role model means to you? Consider confidence and leadership.

It is about understanding other people and showing up, shining and being visible as the best person and nurse you can be at that particular point in time. It means listening to other people as well as talking, it is about appropriate communication (Kline, 2002). It is not about being perfect and always getting things right. It relates to helping other people and encouraging them to develop and grow, as you have developed and grown professionally. This is because when you are not there, you want to know the work is going to carry on being completed in your absence. If you are going to be someone that people look up to as a role model then you need to know it is okay to admit that you do not know everything, providing you know where your resources are that you can find the answer out from. Knowing who or where to turn to when there is an issue, is more helpful than trying to know everything. For example, if you are working in clinical practice, there is usually a whole myriad of resources such as specialist nurses, specialist people from Allied health medical professions, physiotherapists, dieticians, speech and language therapists, occupational therapists, radiographers, to name but a few. These people may know the answers to questions or it may be appropriate for them to undertake work rather than you.

Being the best you can be at work is about being positive and it is about being professional and promoting trust (NMC, 2015). Whilst we all have colleagues who do not do things the way we would do them, it is acknowledging that their way might still be safe and acceptable. Explaining why you do things differently and discussing differences in approaches facilitates both sides learning (Elock & Sharples, 2011). This would either be at the time if it is appropriate or taking them to one side at a later time. Use suitable ways of communication for explaining to people and giving them information about how things should be done if you do not think they are being done in a correct manner. Particularly if there seems to be something unsafe, or very close to unsafe behaviour or practice. It is about having boundaries, principles and standards that you maintain, so that people know the expectations of performance at work. Show up as yourself by behaving consistently as people will then trust you.

Exercise 17. Write notes about what being a mentor means to you. If you are a qualified mentor, discuss with other mentors how you achieve effective mentorship in your work.

Mentoring – feedback. Relevant points 1.1, 1.3, 7.1, 7.4, 7.5, 8, 9.1, 9.4, 11, 20.8 (NMC, 2015).

References
Bradbury L (Ed) (2013) *The F Factor.* CreateSpace Independent Publishing Platform.
Dickson A (2015) *A woman in your own right: assertiveness and you.* Quartet Books
Earvolino-Ramirez (2007) *Resilience a concept analysis.* Nursing Forum 42(2) Apr-Jun: 72-83.
Elock K and Sharples K (2011) *A Nurse's Survival Guide to Mentoring* London. Churchill Livingston Elsevier.
Gray J (2012) *Building resilience in the workforce* (Editorial) Nursing Standard 26(32) Apr 11: 1.

Hart P, Brannan JD & De Chesnay M (2014) *Resilience in nurses: an integrative review* Journal of Nursing Management 22: 720-734.

NMC (2015) *Code of Conduct.* London. NMC.

Pegram A & Bloomfield J (2015) *Nutrition and fluid management* Nursing Standard 29(31) 1-7 Apr: 38-42.

Kline N (2002) *Time to think. Listening to ignite the human mind* London. Cassell.

NMC (2015) *Code of Conduct.* London. NMC.

Redgrave S & Townsend N (2005) *You can win at life! Unlock your potential and go for gold...* London. BBC Books.

Richardson C (2009) *The art of extreme self-care: transform your life one month at a time.* London. Hay House.

Trueland J (2016) *The many benefits of 'always events'.* Nursing Standard 30(22) Jan27-Feb2: 24-25.

Wicks RJ (2005) *Overcoming secondary stress in medical and nursing practice: a guide to professional resilience and personal well-being.* Oxford. Oxford University Press.

www.NurseRevalidationBook.co.uk

Chapter 6
The art and science within the registered nurse

Utilising your masculine and feminine systems

Discussion about the art and science of nursing is not new, however I want you to consider the art and science within you. The majority of people have a mix of masculine and feminine traits. Knowing when it is right to use one or the other, or a combination of the two is a skill to cultivate. Recognising your own masculine and feminine traits is a precursor to understanding how to use them wisely (Bradbury, 2013).

There has been a tendency to equate art with feminine traits and characteristics and science with masculine traits and characteristics. Avoid making assumptions that males are naturally more scientific or females are more creative ('arty').

In my experience, art in nursing is about creativity broadly speaking, not specifically drawing or painting. Qualitative research and new ways of providing services to the public are commonly creative. The majority of nurses I have encountered have been highly creative. They have been working in situations with; limited resources, equipment, staffing, people who are challenging to manage (either patients, relatives and/or staff), and they do a lot of reflection in action to quickly create the right circumstance for somebody to get the best possible nursing care that they can, at that point, be given. That may be safe nursing care and is the best available at that time, which is acceptable. [See Diagram 1, Chapter 5.]

Measurement is scientific, for example, measuring observations, respiratory rate, oxygen saturations, heart rate, capillary refill (central or peripheral), Blood Pressure, temperature, weight, height are part of clinical practice. Statistics and audit of bed occupancy, number of operations performed, number of admissions from the Emergency Department are also measurements. Quantitative Research is based on use of measureable variables. Technology might be considered as science and it encompasses completing charts, using the telephone, using computers, operating complicated intravenous fluid machines or cardiac monitors.

Are your characteristics more art or science, or an equal mix?	
Write your art characteristics:	Write your science characteristics:
[For example: people watching and imagining their life stories; making things...]	[For example: organising meetings; calculating statistics...]
How can these help you with your reflections? In what way do you use them effectively in your daily work?	How can these assist you with your planning? In which ways do you use them effectively in your daily work?
Relate these to any of the relevant points in the NMC (2015) Code of Conduct	
	Exercise 18

Creative communication

Exercise 19. Consider how you use creative communication in your work. Write a list of how you do this.

Your communication at work is about being skilled at giving information verbally, non-verbally and also receiving information. Being aware of the wide range of ways you can use non-verbal communication and the effect these have on others. It is not just about body language, is also about tone and pitch of the voice, speed at which you speak, posture and how you present yourself, eye contact, touch, using your senses (although smell and taste are not normally part of communication). If you are involved in working with people with cognitive impairment or children and young people, it might involve play perhaps combined with drawing or use of pictures. Distress can cause people to function or communicate in different ways, not normally. Aiming to de-stress people can improve their cognitive ability and they may be better able to listen and take in what you are saying, because they are less worried about themselves and/or their relatives.

If you are an educator or manager, it might also be about how you get your message across to your other staff. A sense of fun is important but humour must be used in a positive and playful way, where people can easily understand it is being used as jesting and not as unpleasant banter nor a way to make fun of someone in a negative way.

Speaking, using similarities or common terms can be extremely helpful, however it is important to make sure people understand them. Particularly in education, using popular expressions that are common in English, people from other countries particularly if English is not their first language may find these difficult to understand. It might be better to begin with explaining the cultural norms of the UK and cultural differences.

Points 1 or 2 are relating to communication and points 7.1 to 7.5 are also relevant. (NMC, 2015).

Exercise 20. How do you use humour at work? Write notes on how you ensure that people understand your correct intention of comedy. You could ask co-workers how they interpret, understand and appreciate your sense of humour.

Creative performance

You are you and you are enough (Bradbury, 2013). Introduce yourself with "I am <your name>" followed by "I am the nurse who will be looking after you today" (Grainger, 2013). Being a nurse is a role, a part of your life, it does not define you. The nurse as a role is in some ways like being an actor. Acting is creative performance, because you may go to work with physical, emotional or social issues you are worrying about and/or are at the back of your mind that mean being a nurse might feel difficult today. Although you may be convinced you need to go to work and you need to perform in a safe manner.

Creative performance is required without the high drama! But be authentic (human) and putting part of yourself into the interaction, as generally people respond positively to that (Bradbury, 2013). Then you will receive feedback about your performance (chapter 2).

The nurse acts confidently despite how they feel, it is not about acting competent when you are not competent, it is knowing the limits and being responsible for your actions. Being confident is particularly important in terms of gaining trust from other people, they need to trust the nurse. They want the nurse (you) to be able to convince them they can look after them satisfactorily. They are putting their whole trust into the health system and you represent that system.

Creative performance is about showing up, not as yourself only but as yourself the nurse - whatever that means to you (chapter 1). Part of your creative performance is dressing as the professional nurse, by adhering to their organisation's dress code, which have been developed with infection-control, moving and handling, and safety issues in mind to protect the nurse's physical safety. Dressing as the professional is part of the creative performance before work commences, including neat and tidy hair to assist in infection control. [Points 19.3, 19.4 & 20 (NMC, 2015)]

Creative performance is also about managing your emotions. There will be situations which may make you want to cry, laugh or scream, although it is not appropriate to in the situation. How you manage those emotions will affect others around you.

Measuring knowledge and career development

This is related to knowing your professional purpose and measuring how far along the journey you have travelled. What promises and intentions have you achieved already? Which ones are left to complete? (Redgrave & Townsend, 2005, Bradbury, 2013)

Successfully completing courses can measure your knowledge, but it is not the sole way to do so. Competence is a way to measure knowledge and skill acquisition (see the next section). In clinical practice using the Knowledge and Skills Framework (KSF) allows benchmarking and then tracking of progress (DH, 2004).

Updating your Curriculum Vitae (CV) [Chapter 8] can demonstrate your accomplishments to date. Additionally, so can completing your annual personal development review or appraisal.

Use your science characteristics to discover how to measure your knowledge and your career development.

Continuing professional development is your simple route to revalidation. Revisit the information you wrote in Chapter 3 and re-evaluate your time-line. If things are going to plan, then you can continue on the same trajectory. If dates have been missed, then take into consideration why this has occurred. Make decisions about the assistance you might need to get back on track and pick the relevant people and resources to best assist you.

Spend time looking inward and discovering why you have been unable to keep your promises to yourself, as without this knowledge you may simply keep making the same mistakes without learning from them. (Richardson, 2009, Holt, 2012 & Dickson, 2015)

Measuring competence

This can be in terms of skills achieved, for example, once you have qualified, there will be additional skills that make you competent to do your job that were not part of the student nurse role. Competence occurs in point 13 (NMC, 2015).

The theory relating to additional skills is usually taught at study sessions and then you have to be supervised in practice until you are deemed safe and competent in these skills. There are often booklets or forms that require signing off by other competent nurses who have clinically supervised you. The example form is an overview framework again, providing clarity of ease to look at, to show to prospective employers at interviews, and also to your confirmer to demonstrate your progress.

Example form to capture skills you have become competent in.

Skills competence	Date signed as competent	Re-assessment date (if required):
Medications administration		
IV Medications administration		
Venepuncture		
Cannulation		
Naso-Gastric (NG) tube placement		
Naso-Gastric (NG) tube feeding		
Wound closure		
Breaking bad news		
Blood gas machine use		
Giving verbal and written information to patients		
Life support: Basic, Immediate, Advanced [adult or child or neonatal]		
Giving feedback to students who are failing or who have failed		
Presenting at internal or external University Examination Boards		
Delivering a report or paper to a Trust Board		
Presenting at a curriculum revalidation		

Form 4

Exercise 21. List the competences that you have successfully completed on your own form.

References

Argyle M (1994) *The Psychology of Interpersonal Behaviour.* 5th Ed. Harmondsworth. Penguin.

Bradbury L (Ed) (2013) *The F Factor.* CreateSpace Independent Publishing Platform.

Department of Health (2004) *The Knowledge and Skills Framework (NHS KSF) and the Development Review Process.* London. Department of Health.

Dickson A (2015) *A woman in your own right: assertiveness and you.* London. Quartet Books.

Granger K (2013) *Hello, my name is... campaign.*

Holt L (2012) *Get out of your own way. Stop sabotaging your business and learn to stand out in a crowded market.* London. National Alliance of Business Owners.

NMC (2015) *Code of Conduct.* London. NMC.

Redgrave S & Townsend N (2005) *You can win at life! Unlock your potential and go for gold...* London. BBC Books.

Richardson C (2009) *The art of extreme self-care: transform your life one month at a time.* London. Hay House.

Chapter 7
The reflective registered nurse

Look inward

The reflective nurse takes personal responsibility and looks inward. Looking inward might not seem to be the easiest thing in the world to do, but the NMC wants us to be reflective practitioners. Be proactive and find out, or remind yourself, what a reflective practitioner is all about and how you do reflection.

Reflection is also about self-knowledge and self-development, thinking not just about one part of you but holistically [body, mind and spirit]. It is also considering whether or not you are going to do an individual reflection or you are going to use individual reflection coupled with how the team works, or you will decide to undertake reflection looking solely at teamwork.

It can be more difficult focusing specifically on teamwork because you are always going to reflect on what you are doing. Balanced reflection is important as it is about looking at the positive and negative things that have happened when reflecting, not focusing solely on one aspect. Although the NMC suggests focusing on positives (NMC,

2016a). Your reflection may be on something unusual or on more common and frequent occurrences.

In 3 years, the NMC are only expecting 5 reflective pieces, which is less than 2 per year. These must be documented on the forms they have developed and the link is on my website. You may wish to reflect more often, in order to continue learning and developing professionally. Consider identifying regular time in your work diary to choose an incident to reflect on. This might be 1 day every 3 months. If it is not your preferred learning style, you may decide to do less reflection and more of the other types of knowledge acquisition, such as reading or online quizzes.

Exercise 22. For your reflection you will need to:

- Make brief notes at the time. If you need to refer back to patient or student notes, then keep a record of the actual name, but in a safe place at work to ensure their confidentiality is maintained.
- Contemplate, and write down, what you want to gain from this reflection.
- Think how this reflection might enable you to improve in the future.
- Consider who would benefit from you sharing your reflection with them. You may wish to talk about it with your reflective discussion partner first.
(Rogers & Freiburg, 1994)

- Allocate time in your diary to undertake the process of reflection.
- Use resources that are evidence based to discover if there is literature that is new to you.

Be honest with yourself (Baretta, 2014) when you use the reflective process. This does not require you to judge yourself or others' actions negatively, merely to describe how the incident occurred in a factual way (NMC, 2016a).

For updates visit: www.NurseRevalidationBook.co.uk

Models for reflection

There are a number of models for reflection, for example: Schön (1984), Gibbs (1988), Johns (2009). You may have already used one and find it suitable. Otherwise, I suggest you read the models and decide which one you will feel most comfortable using. Although you could try all of them on different pieces of reflection if you wish, since you may find you prefer using one more than the others. Whatever works best for you, if you find one model is too complicated then try using another one. Avoid a 'mix and match' approach, by resisting using parts from different models of reflection in one of your reflective pieces as this may prove too confusing.

In terms of how you structure your reflection, the majority of the reflective models use a cyclical process, providing a framework on which to base your reflection. Point 6.1 relates to reflection (NMC, 2015).

Look at why the models were written and developed and review the books about them. This may entail you reading the whole book or you may simply skim-read the book, then take the framework they use and see if you can make sense of the model yourself. Depending on the sort of learner you are articles may be easier to read than a book. Articles are obviously shorter than a book and the author of the article may have provided examples of how they themselves have used the model they are writing about.

The models should help you review the situation with ease, if you are finding it difficult then you may have to reconsider whether or not it is the best model for you. Trying a different model may be more appropriate.

Exercise 23. Consider the models and make an informed choice about which 1 might suit you best.

Reflection in action

Reflection in action is about being in the moment and changing what you are doing because you are reflecting on what you are actually doing. For example, something might not be going as well as you wanted it to and you realise it immediately, you think about how you might change things and carry out the action to do so.

One illustration is when I was a Sister in an emergency department. I was standing up with my arms crossed, talking to a patient who had taken an overdose of drugs, which were potentially lethal, and he needed to stay in hospital for treatment. He was standing opposite me wearing only a hospital gown and was very agitated, he was also slightly shorter than me or a similar height. I was explaining to him how important it was that he stayed in hospital for treatment and that we wanted to help him, because he was insistent he wanted to go home. I realised during this interaction that I had my arms crossed, and as I had recently attended a communication course when I had been told that crossed arms represented a barrier and makes people think you are either in control of them or angry towards them. Essentially it comes across as negative, non-verbal communication. (Argyle, 1988 & 1994). Slowly, without doing anything obvious, I uncrossed my arms and let my arms hang by my sides whilst carrying on talking in an encouraging tone of voice saying exactly the same things I had previously been saying. Repeating how important it was for him to stay in hospital and get the correct treatment. Within a couple of minutes of my uncrossing my arms and changing my posture this young man calmed down then said "yes sister" and went back to his cubicle.

Another instance was when I was teaching to a mixture of students, many of whom did not speak English as their first language. I used the phrase "nowt so queer as folk" to describe the feelings I had of people's unexpected behaviour, and as I looked at the faces of my students they showed no signs of understanding. I realised I had used an English saying that held no meaning for them. By instantly rewording the phrase, the whole group were able to understand what I meant.

Therefore, reflection in action can be a really powerful consideration by thinking about actions as they take place and recognising the need to change some aspect of what you are doing, immediately.

Reflection in action links with creative communication and creative performance that were considered in chapter 6. It is about bringing love and light to every situation, but avoiding getting caught up in unnecessary drama (Bradbury, 2013).

Exercise 24. What reflection in action have you undertaken in your daily practice today? Reflect on its effectiveness.

Reflection on action

This is the more common type of reflection and it is used retrospectively. Taking time after work to look back on the actions that were taken during the day and reflect on them. It is consideration of the actions that occurred in the past. There is a risk that our memory will not remember actions accurately or an element of judgement will enter the reflection made in hindsight. These are aspects to be aware of but should not be a bar to undertaking reflection. Reflections can be used to encourage and not to judge (Bradbury, 2013) or to use constructive, objective, and professional judgement, if appropriate.

Reflection is about considering what has been done, did it work well and could it have worked better? Is there anything that you would do in the future to change how you might react in a similar situation? Is it an experience that might happen again? If it did take place again would you act the same or do something differently? If you did something in a particular way, is there evidence in the literature that says this particular way works best? Thinking about it and asking if it did actually work best in this instance?

Sometimes there is research evidence that says doing X in Y way will work best, but actually in the situation in which you found yourself, because health care is very complex, possibly X did not work for you in the Y situation. You can consider what the research and evidence theory was, although in the situation that you found yourself in, you did something different because it worked better. With consideration, think about what would you replicate in the future or would you try what the evidence suggested and see whether or not that works in a different situation? Use a model as your framework (see chapter 7).

It is also about having confidence in yourself to make those kinds of decisions. Reflection is generally undertaken by individuals, but in terms of requiring participatory study hours (Chapter 3) it would be a helpful idea to do reflection as a group or team as well. This is often termed 'debriefing'. A short informal 'debrief' of 10-15 minutes may be as valuable as a 1 hour formal 'debrief', particularly if all the team members are encouraged to speak (Kline, 2002).

Time any discussion in order for it to count as part of your participatory study time. Those are the 20 hours that you need to complete over 3 years.

Exercise 25. Write a piece of reflection, using the NMC form. Meet with your Reflective Discussion Partner or confirmer to discuss it.

Balanced reflection

The thing about using a reflective model is getting some balance and avoid just focussing on the negatives. NMC wants positive reflections, expecting nurses to recognise there are so many good things that happen in the healthcare service every day, that often get overlooked, missed or forgotten (NMC, 2016a). Within the healthcare service, it is very common for healthcare professionals to only look at complaints and mistakes and what went wrong, although it is important to learn from all those things you also need to look at the positive situations and what went right. It is then looking at what would be good to replicate in the future.

There are 2 reasons for this:

1. You can learn from something that went right and ensure you incorporate it into future practice. The things you know to do well and the things that work. Also, you communicate that within the team.
2. Focusing on positive things makes you feel much better. Positive reflection increases your motivation to go to work, it makes you feel good and confident. There are things that you get right at work and you can actually achieve.

There is much literature written about personal development and relating to the resilience of staff and their recommendations are to focus on what is going right. (Richardson, 2009; Wicks, 2005). The society that we live in has a very negative focus. Switching the news on means being bombarded with negative events with very little good news to balance it out and make people feel good about themselves. At the end of your working day, if something has gone wrong and it might only be one small thing that's gone wrong in that day, it is common that people will often focus on the one negative thing and say they have had a really bad day because one thing did not go right. And that can be really demoralising. Instead, try thinking about gratitude:

- Did someone say thank you?

Was someone really pleased you were able to do something for them that worked really well? It might be a patient or their relative if you are a clinical front-line nurse, it might be one of your staff if you are a manager, or it could be a student if you're an educationalist. Try to remember at least 5 positive aspects of your day [Wicks 2005]. This may also provide you with feedback evidence and you require 5 types of feedback in 3 years (NMC, 2016a).

Exercise 26. Be grateful when things go right at work, smile at and praise staff too.

To err is human

Making mistakes and learning from them is important. A vital thing to remember is 'to err is human', we all make mistakes, but making a mistake is not necessarily a bad thing. Learning from our mistakes sometimes it makes us better at doing whatever it is we need to do. For example, from an inventor - Edison and his light bulb, he got one to work properly after trying 180 or more and someone asked, 'how did it feel to make all those mistakes?' Edison apparently replied, 'they weren't mistakes they were just versions of light bulbs that didn't work properly until I got to the one that did.' Trial and error and perseverance are important.

In the UK, it seems there is a drive to eliminate risk in the health service and the culture implies that people should not make mistakes, despite rhetoric encouraging healthcare professionals to report errors. That is unrealistic and although in a healthcare profession, particularly in clinical practice, making a mistake can be something that causes the death of a patient, nonetheless making one mistake is seldom life-threatening in itself. It is more commonly a series of errors, made by more than one healthcare professional.

Life is inherently risky and death is the end result for 100% of the world's population. Risk reduction is the best that can be planned for.

When you are working in a team, just because one person makes a mistake it is likely that someone in the team will notice it allowing remedial action to be taken. On occasion, patient deterioration has been missed by several staff members, hence the introduction of the Acute Life-threatening Events Recognition and Treatment (ALERT) course (ALERT, 1999) and the National Early Warning Score (Royal College of Physicians, 2015) to reduce the risk of similar events.

The focus was on 'Never events' and avoiding harm. Now there is increasing emphasis on 'Always events', which are an action-oriented set of behaviours that clearly foster partnering with patients and their relatives, it exhibits a sustained family-centred care style and established enriched outcomes and optimum experience for the patient plus meeting the 4 criteria of: importance; measurable; evidence-based; sustainable and affordable. (NHS England, 2015, Trueland, 2016). Learning has happened as the focus is moving from mistakes to prevention (see also Chapter 5). Embrace our imperfections (Bradbury, 2013) and shine, plus learn from them.

Exercise 27. Makes notes about how you feel about making mistakes? Can you still feel confident afterwards?

References
Acute Life-threatening Events Recognition and Treatment (ALERT) (1999)
Argyle M (1988) *Bodily communication.* Routledge.
Argyle M (1994) *The psychology of interpersonal behaviour.* 5th Ed. Harmondsworth. Penguin.
Baratta S (2014) *Simple Success. In business and in life.* Willow Tree 3.
Bradbury L (Ed) (2013) *The F Factor.* CreateSpace Independent Publishing Platform.
Gibbs G (1988) *Learning by doing. A guide to teaching and learning methods.* FEU.

Johns C (2009) *Becoming a reflective practitioner.* 3rd Ed. Wiley Blackwell. Chichester.

Kline N (2002) *Time to think. Listening to ignite the human mind.* London. Cassell.

NHS England (2015) *Building the right support.* NHS. London.

NMC (2015) *Code of Conduct.* London. NMC.

NMC (2016a) *Revalidation. How to revalidate with the NMC.* Requirements for renewing your registration. London. NMC.

Richardson C (2009) *The art of extreme self-care: transform your life one month at a time.* London. Hay House.

Rogers C & Freiberg HJ (1994) *Freedom to learn.* 3rd Ed. London. Prentice Hall.

Royal College of Physicians (2015) *National Early Warning Score. Standardising the assessment of acute-illness severity in the NHS.* London.

Schön D (1984) *The reflective practitioner. How professionals think in action.* Basic Books.

Trueland J (2016) *The many benefits of 'always events'.* Nursing Standard 30(22) Jan27-Feb2: 24-25.

Wicks RJ (2005) *Overcoming secondary stress in medical and nursing practice: a guide to professional resilience and personal well-being.* Oxford. Oxford University Press.

www.NurseRevalidationBook.co.uk

Chapter 8
Owning your portfolio

Fill up first

Owning your portfolio might seem like a strange statement. The NMC (2015) does not mandate that registered nurses must keep a portfolio, but it seems eminently sensible to do so. The portfolio may be paper or electronic format. If you choose not to use a portfolio, then you need to think of another way of keeping and organising the evidence you need for your CPD and revalidation.

The point about 'owning it' is acknowledging that it is your responsibility to fill it up and it is your property. You have to hold yourself accountable for keeping it up to date and for ensuring it is in a safe place and for keeping back-up copies of anything important. It is not up to your confirmer or your reflective discussion partner to do any of the above, they are simply people who will assist you in your revalidation process. If they are willing, they can help you keep yourself accountable. You would have to ask them.

If you choose to have a portfolio, then you need to take responsibility for obtaining evidence, putting information in to your portfolio, sorting out the order in your portfolio, and making your portfolio look professional.

Since your evidence for revalidation demonstrates your continuing professional development, this is something that you will take to job interviews as well as your appraisal (personal development review). When attending an interview or your personal development review, print off two or three portfolio entries, for the interviewers/reviewer, which demonstrates your capability to do the job. They should ask to look at your portfolio, so this will demonstrate preparation and save them having to find examples in a large portfolio.

Another aspect of obtaining evidence is about timing and how long it is going to take. Work out how long will it take you to write a reflective piece. Decide how many reflective pieces are you going to be doing – the minimum of 5 required by NMC or more? (NMC, 2016a) (See chapter 8). Never underestimate how much time it is going to take, it is important to allocate time in your diary to do this.

Even if you are a deadline person, plan this as it continuing professional development. Organising evidence and collating it maybe last minute, but you will already have all the information that you require. The focus is that this is activity over time and speaking with reflective discussion partners and/or confirmers must take place. It will be impossible to leave revalidation until the night before your registration expires.

As a word of caution, there is now a lengthy process to re-register if your registration lapses and you will be unable to work during this time.

For further updates: www.NurseRevalidationBook.co.uk

Curriculum Vitae

There are 3 reasons why it is important to have a curriculum vitae (CV).

1) In order for you to summarise your achievements in one place.
2) To enable you to appreciate your incredible achievements.
3) To be prepared for your next opportunity or job application.

Your CV is a chance for you to review your career progress and your achievements. Writing them down makes them visible, allowing you to congratulate yourself, which can be highly motivating.

Have a CV prepared because you never know when a job or opportunity might come up and if you're looking to progress you should always be looking towards enhancing your career development. Organisations, such as the Florence Nightingale Foundation, offer scholarships with finance to enable you to develop, find the link at the website for this book.

Claire Picton

By reading this book you are demonstrating that you care about your registration and therefore about nursing.

Example layout for CV

Your name		
Your contact details		
Your employer and their contact details.		
Summary of who you are (brief) *I am a credible and motivational RN who has the opportunities to learn and develop throughout her career and pass on knowledge to colleagues in a professional leadership role... The experience as the Consultant Nurse... My experience as the Journal editor... The time when I was committee member of RCN ECA and Council member of Shared Interest gave... As an active Christian, I understand that the spiritual dimension... I have maintained academic links with... I believe that the above will...*		
Referee 1 Role & contact details:		Referee 2 Role & contact details:
Your current job title:		Date commenced:
Outline of responsibilities of role		
Academic Qualifications		
Date obtained:	Qualification gained:	Awarding Institution:
Clinical courses attended:		
Membership of professional organisations:		
Date of entry:	Organisation:	Number:
	Nursing & Midwifery Council	
	Royal College of Nursing	
Previous Employment		
Dates:	Post held and the organisation's name:	Very brief outline of responsibilities:
Volunteer roles:		
Dates:	Organisation's Name:	Activities undertaken:
Publications. *[Letter(s) to journal; article; report; book chapter; book.]*		
Author(s):	Year of publication:	Title and reference:
Presentations. *[Within your organisation; at your local University; regionally; nationally; internationally. Speak in the debating session at RCN Congress.]*		
Non-nursing and/or volunteering. *[Completed Duke of Edinburgh Award – Bronze, Silver &/or Gold. 'Head of Household' – managing a home and raising a child, caring for elders.]*		
National work/volunteering.		
International work/volunteering.		
Consultancy Work/volunteering.		

Even at the beginning of your career you have achievements. Such positive undertakings are great to highlight for job applications. To be successful you have to take action, demonstrating you are going beyond your remit. This will make you stand out from others.

For further updates visit: www.NurseRevalidationBook.co.uk

Gathering evidence and storing it for easy retrieval

Looking at evidence from the viewpoint for nurses in clinical practice, it is easy to relate to the Code of Conduct (NMC, 2015) as it is primarily focussed upon nurses who directly care for patients. It is understandable given that patient safety is a priority.

Managers who are nurses, nurse educators and nurses who wish to retain their registration but do not directly care for the general public will be looking for different types of evidence. Education manager roles may share similarities with general manager roles.

Prioritising people will be about staff, for managers. Points 1.1; 1.3; 1.5; 2.2; 2.6; 3.1 (NMC, 2015) appear to be applicable to staff.

Exercise 28. The health of staff is vital to ensure they are fit for duty. As a leader what is your responsibility in relation to point 3.1 (NMC, 2015)? How do you positively:

- Promote well-being?
- Prevent ill health?

Those employed as senior lecturers in a University, you will be mainly involved with undergraduate or postgraduate students.

Exercise 29. What do you do in terms of:

- Personal development for those students, what sort of tutorial support do you provide?
- Curriculum development - how you manage and structure your courses, how you deliver your seminars and lectures?
- Supporting your peers?

Which points in the Code of Conduct (NMC, 2015) do the above answers relate to?

Easy retrieval of evidence is important for times when you may be able to have an impromptu discussion with your reflective discussion partner or confirmer. Is there a safe place to keep a paper-based portfolio in your workplace? Electronic storage is increasingly the quickest retrieval method, but may be difficult for those who find information technology and use of computers challenging. Having backup copies of all your evidence is prudent so it can be produced on demand, since the NMC still intends to randomly pick registrants and review their evidence (NMC (2016a).

Reflective discussion for those nurses who need to go outside of their department where they work or external to their organisation to undertake peer-to-peer discussion, if their confirmer is a non-nurse, will require evidence that is easily portable.

Documentation

There is the requirement to keep clear and accurate records relevant to your practice (NMC, 2015) and revalidation evidence links with this. Points 10.5 & 10.6 seem particularly relevant (NMC, 2015).

Ensure you use the documents that the NMC requires. There is a guidance document that you need to read completely and the NMC (2016a) has produced various forms that need to be completed in order to successfully revalidate. I strongly advise that you familiarise yourself with these. The links are on the website linked with this book. I suggest that a copy the NMC code of conduct (2015) is kept in your portfolio, so that it is at hand when you need to reference it.

In terms of documentation, there are many national documents, legislation or guidance that you work according to. For those who practice in England the six Cs are principles and a framework you can utilise in practice. The six Cs are: care, compassion, competence, communication, courage and commitment (Cummings, 2012). For those working in social care, Skills for Care have devised the Social Care Commitment, which provides another framework to guide your evidence gathering (link is on the website associated with this book). The Knowledge Skills Framework can be useful for those working under Agenda for Change (DH, 2004, see also Chapter 6).

To make life easier for your reflective discussion partner and/or confirmer depending on whether they are one or the same person, it is probably a good idea to type rather than hand write. When you show your reflective pieces to your reflective discussion partner (RDP) and/or confirmer try and give it to them before your meeting date. This provides them an opportunity to read them in advance in order to maximise the amount of time you have to talk about your reflections. This provides them the opportunity to think about relevant questions to ask you. The NMC also suggests this is good practice for the nurse RDP and/or nurse confirmer to learn about the revalidation process if they have not yet undertaken on their own.

Exercise 30. Negotiate dates to meet with your RDP and/or confirmer and schedule them in your diary. Additionally, book the date for your yearly review with your Line Manager and include that in your diary as soon as you can.

Archiving

You need to know what you have to have in your portfolio or as evidence. The requirement for the NMC is that you have 3 years of information and evidence, anything that is more than 3 years old needs be archived (NMC, 2016a). The exceptions are: if it is a once only course that will be valid for the whole of your nursing career. For example, your initial nurse education becoming an RGN will be valid for the whole of your life in terms of that qualification, you can put that into your portfolio or evidence file. Some courses are always valid, but do need regular updates.

Your original certificates can be photocopied if you are keeping your portfolio as a paper copy or scan them into an electronic portfolio.

Example sections for your portfolio: Reflection. Feedback. Knowledge and skills framework (KSF) criteria. 6Cs standards. Social Care Commitment standards. Courses. Statutory and Mandatory courses. Study Days. Curriculum Vitae. NMC Code of Conduct.

Exercise 31. What other sections would be appropriate for your portfolio?

If you are keeping your portfolio in a public place, such as at work, it is more sensible to put in a copy of your certificate(s) in your portfolio as you will need to keep your original(s) in a safe place. That will probably be at home and if you have a safe then you may wish to keep them in there. Or you may wish to frame them and to display them. The choice is yours. There may be other courses you do not need to update, for example your original mentorship course or the Postgraduate certificate in educating adults, or equivalent, would not need updating. Although you would need to do a mentor update, which is an add-on to your original course.

Do you need to keep your portfolio information and evidence if it is older than three years? It is up to you to make the decision. If you are the sort of person that likes to keep hold of that information, then the answer is obviously yes. I suggest you put it into different file or folder as an archive. Otherwise it can be archived into the rubbish bin, shredded or recycled. However, before you recycle it, as in the section on your CV, be sure to capture the information within your CV. Otherwise you might forget things. As said previously, it is about being able to reflect back on all the positives you have done and appreciate your awesomeness. Personal responsibility for making a decision whether to keep information or not is yours.

Keeping it live

Your evidence is your tool for learning and developing yourself, it demonstrates your Continuing Professional Development (CPD). It shows self-care and that you value yourself.

Keeping it live follows on from archiving. The key points and, again going back to personal responsibility, but also about time management and planning is to ensure you are adding to your portfolio on at least a monthly basis. I suggest putting small pieces of information and evidence in on a weekly basis. It depends on the busyness of your life and what you can realistically achieve. Make it something that is achievable. As stated previously, promise yourself you are going to do it, schedule it in your diary so that you know what you are going to be doing and when you're going to be doing it. When you work make sure you make notes of things that are really important for you to be able to reflect on them for your portfolio evidence.

I cannot tell you exactly how much to do as it is very personal, although you need to achieve the requirements of the NMC (2016a). What I can suggest is that you make a decision about what you're going to do and wherever possible you keep to that. Things will change from month-to-month because your personal circumstances and workload will alter.

This is not about revalidation taking over your life. Have a life, you need a life, get a life. Work is not all of your existence, it is only a small part of you. And it does not define you.

It is about keeping your professional confidence live, and you convincing yourself that you can re-register as a nurse with ease. It also helps you to see you are achieving things and making progress.

Avoid people who waste time and energy moaning and/or who are full of negatives. Pick people who can help you, ask other people what they have done and pick people with high energy and a positive can-do attitude. Find people who positively want to embrace developing themselves and progressing and learning. Know who those people are, you will feel different around them, they will want to be improving themselves and to be joyful in doing so. That is the sort of person you need to be around to actually increase your energy and get you enthused.

Exercise 32 . How would you keep your CPD and portfolio live? What is it that you need to do? Write these things down and schedule them in your diary otherwise they will not happen. If you put it in your diary and but are unable to achieve it, simply reschedule it – do not beat yourself up because you have not done it, accept that changes sometimes need to be made. Re-evaluate whether there is still a need to do it. Make yourself promises because if you do not break promises to other people, you should not break promises to yourself. Love yourself (Richardson, 2009).

References
Cummings J (2012) *Compassion in Practice. Nursing, midwifery and care staff. Our vision for the future.* Department of Health. London.
Department of Health (2004) *The Knowledge and Skills Framework (NHS KSF) and the Development Review Process.* London. Department of Health.

NMC (2015) *Code of Conduct.* London. NMC.

NMC (2016a) *Revalidation. How to revalidate with the NMC. Requirements for renewing your registration.* London. NMC.

Richardson C (2009) *The art of extreme self-care: transform your life one month at a time.* London. Hay House.

www.NurseRevalidationBook.co.uk

Chapter 9
Removing drama from the lives of registered nurses

NMC Code of Conduct (2015)

The NMC (2015) Code of Conduct is a standard and framework that governs our practice as nurses. There are four main sections in the Code of Conduct and they are further divided into detailed points. It assists in removing unnecessary drama from the lives of registered nurses. The idea with the new revalidation process is that we refer to it frequently. It is up to us to decide what period of regularity - daily, weekly or monthly. This is because as part of our continuing professional development we have to weave strands of the Code of Conduct through our revalidation process. The introduction to the code gives more information (NMC, 2016a).

Chapter 6 considered drama as a positive creative performance and relinquishing unnecessary drama, which is when we hype things up and get them out of all proportion. The standards and behaviours are detailed in the Code of Conduct for nurses to refer to and use. It is visible for the general public, and members of the multidisciplinary team, to reference, so that they know what expectations they can have of nurses as professionals. (NMC, 2015).

Interpretation of the Code of Conduct

Putting patients first is very commendable, but the UK needs nurses who are not only fit for purpose but also who are fit to work. If nurses do not take care of their own needs first and prioritise themselves, preserve their own safety and trust themselves, then they will not be in the best state to care for others. (Wicks, 2005) Point 20.9 (NMC, 2015)

Educators should be guiding and educating nurses about resilience and self-care (Richardson, 2009; Wicks, 2005) Managers have a responsibility to ensure that good practice occurs and that staff are taking breaks during their shifts and reporting to their managers if this is not happening. Nurses' health and well-being has often come second and the consequence is that managers then have to 'manage' high sickness levels. Healthy food choices in the staff restaurant, opportunities to relax in a staff room that is a pleasant environment, a chance to take physical activity (for example, walking outside, whacking a SwingBall™ about); sitting in a pleasant, secluded staff garden could be available in all healthcare organisations. There are employers who have provided such facilities.

Occupational Health departments and their staff often work with healthcare staff about their sickness. Consistently focussing on prevention of ill-health, self-care and resilience in staff would be more proactive.

The next sections will consider how the Code of Conduct relates to revalidation with ease. In other words, how you can make revalidation easeful for you.

Prioritise people

Looking at the Code of Conduct, it is clearly written for people who are using midwifery or nursing services to safeguard them. This Code of Conduct can also be interpreted as relating to how nurses should be caring for themselves and their peers, in order to be 'fit' to practice. Point 20.9 states you should keep yourself 'healthy' in order to practise as a nurse.

Exercise 33. What is your definition of healthy? Do you consider yourself to be healthy at this point in time? If yes, what do you need to do to maintain this? If no, how will you change to become 'healthy'? World Health Organisation (WHO, 1948) definition of health …. "Health is a state of complete physical, mental and social well-being and not merely the absence of disease or infirmity."

Do you uphold your own dignity and articulate your needs? Or do you allow others to treat you without dignity? Point 3.1 (NMC, 2015) exhorts nurses to promote well-being. How can we promote professionalism and expect patients to trust us if we clearly don't look after our own well-being? Point 4 (NMC, 2015) states "act in the best interests of people at all times", write down how you can do that for yourself. In a self-care manner, not a selfish way.

Prioritise people	
Standards:	How you will do this for yourself:
1. Treat yourself as an individual and uphold your dignity.	
2. Listen to yourself and respond to your preferences and concerns.	
3. Make sure that your physical, social and psychological needs are assessed and met.	
4. Act in the best interests of yourself at all times.	
5. Respect your right to privacy and confidentiality.	
	Exercise 34

Practise effectively

Look at the Code of Conduct and interpret this in relation to yourself. Working and communicating co-operatively with people who you have a relationship with at home can make incorporating work into your life more easeful. Supportive relationships at home mean less worry for you when you are at work.

Exercise 35. Considering easeful working. Authentic alignment in action, how can you be yourself at home and at work? Dickson (2015) What boundaries do you set to avoid work taking over your life? How do you commit to being fully present and engaged with your precious ones when you are spending time with them? How do you ensure that you can focus exclusively on work when you are paid to be doing that?

Practise effectively	
Standards:	How you will do this for yourself:
1. Always practise in line with the best available evidence.	
2. Communicate clearly.	
3. Work cooperatively.	
4. Share your skill, knowledge and experience for the benefit of yourself and your precious ones.	
5. Keep clear and accurate records relevant to your revalidation.	
6. Be accountable for your revalidation.	

Exercise 36

Preserve safety

Look at the Code of Conduct (NMC, 2015), but how can this be interpreted for you?

Looking after your own health (body, mind and spirit). What does safety feel like to you? How could that be replicated for the staff you meet in your work?

Be observant. Be aware of risks and potential dangers in your workplace. What legislation, policies, protocols or guidelines govern your daily work?

Exercise 37. List what frameworks you use in your daily work that keep you safe:

List the frameworks you use in your daily work that keep you safe:	
Guidance:	How you interpret and use them daily:
Example: Moving and handling legislation [applies to clinicians, managers and educators equally, as it covers moving people and inanimate objects.]	Clinicians: moving and handling inanimate objects such as equipment (pushing trolleys/beds/emergency equipment/machines to measure observations), plus patients. Managers: moving and handling inanimate objects such as equipment, maybe occasionally patients. Educators: carrying equipment to teaching rooms/venues; carrying any physical documents for marking (students' competency documents); carrying photocopying or reams of paper to top up photocopier.
Example: Legislation about safety in the workplace in relation to working hours and taking breaks; the minimum temperature that your employer has to maintain for a comfortable working environment; personal, protective equipment; lone working arrangements (if applicable to you).	

Exercise 37

Promote professionalism and trust

Look at the Code of Conduct (NMC, 2015), but how can this be interpreted?

What does it mean to be a professional? Is it about having a really good knowledge of the evidence that guides your daily practice? Is it about ensuring the reputation of the nursing profession or safeguarding members of the general public? Is it about distance and coldness?

Why and how do you trust people? Why and how do people trust you? How much do you trust yourself? How and when do you replicate that in your daily work to allow the people you work with to trust you? Authentic aligned actions with positive energy, ensuring matching verbal and non-verbal communication assist other people to trust you (Bradbury, 2013).

Promote professionalism and trust.	
Standards:	How you will uphold them for yourself:
1. Uphold the reputation of your profession at all times.	Example: responsible use of social media
2. Uphold your position as a registered nurse or midwife.	Example: in your community, as well as at work
3. Fulfil all registration requirements.	
4. Cooperate with all investigations and audits.	
5. Respond to any complaints made against you professionally.	
6. Provide leadership to make sure people's wellbeing is protected and to improve their experiences of the healthcare system.	

Exercise 38

Integrating the NMC Code of Conduct into daily work

Have the Code of Conduct (NMC, 2015) visible in your work area. Read and become familiar with it. If you are a manager, educator or both and therefore only indirectly affect patient care because you work primarily with staff, then it will mainly be about how you promote it and its values to your students and staff. It should be used to encourage staff.

Study and contemplate what the Code of Conduct means to you and how you can integrate it into your daily practice. Then use the tables below to make notes about how you can use it at work.

You may want to consider whether or not participatory discussions with work colleagues would help your understanding and application of the Code of Conduct (NMC, 2015). It will certainly increase your knowledge of your colleagues' interpretation. Therefore, I suggest talking about it with other nurses will be beneficial. This would also have the advantage of accruing evidence time for your participatory study, but remember to capture the details.

Prioritise people.	
Standards:	How you will uphold them at work:
7. Treat people as individuals and uphold their dignity.	
8. Listen to people and respond to their preferences and concerns.	
9. Make sure that people's physical, social and psychological needs are assessed and responded to.	
10. Act in the best interests of people at all times.	
11. Respect people's right to privacy and confidentiality.	

Exercise 39

Nursing: Your Registration

Practise effectively	
Standards:	How you will uphold them at work:
12. Always practise in line with the best available evidence.	
13. Communicate clearly.	
14. Work cooperatively.	
15. Share your skill, knowledge and experience for the benefit of people receiving care and your colleagues.	
16. Keep clear and accurate records relevant to your practice.	
17. Be accountable for your declaration for decisions to delegate tasks and duties to other people.	
18. Have in place an indemnity arrangement which provides appropriate cover for any practice you take on as a nurse or midwife in the United Kingdom.	
	Exercise 40

Preserve safety	
Standards:	How you will uphold them at work:
19. Recognise and work within the limits of your competence.	
20. Be open and candid with all service users about all aspects of care and treatment, including when any mistakes or harm have taken place.	
21. Always offer help if an emergency arises in your practice setting or anywhere else.	
22. Act without delay if you believe that there is a risk to patient safety or public protection.	
23. Raise concerns immediately if you believe a person is vulnerable or at risk and needs extra support and protection.	
24. Advise on, prescribe, supply, dispense or administer medicines within the limits of your training and competence guidance and other relevant policies, guidance and regulations.	
25. Be aware of, and reduce as far as possible, any potential for harm associated with your practice.	
	Exercise 41

Promote professionalism and trust	
Standards:	How you will uphold them at work:
26. Uphold the reputation of your profession at all times.	
27. Uphold your position as a registered nurse or midwife.	
28. Fulfil all registration requirements.	
29. Cooperate with all investigations and audits.	
30. Respond to any complaints made against you professionally.	
31. Provide leadership to make sure people's wellbeing is protected and to improve their experiences of the healthcare system.	

Exercise 42

If you want to delve deeper into understanding what the NMC (2015) Code of Conduct means in your daily practice and need someone to go through the journey with you, visit the website relating to this book.

References

Bradbury L (Ed) (2013) *The F Factor.* CreateSpace Independent Publishing Platform.

Dickson A (2015) *A woman in your own right: assertiveness and you.* London. Quartet Books.

NMC (2015) *Code of Conduct.* London. NMC.

NMC (2016a) *Revalidation. How to revalidate with the NMC. Requirements for renewing your registration.* London. NMC.

Richardson C (2009) *The art of extreme self-care: transform your life one month at a time.* London. Hay House.

Wicks RJ (2005) *Overcoming secondary stress in medical and nursing practice: a guide to professional resilience and personal well-being.* Oxford. Oxford University Press.

www.NurseRevalidationBook.co.uk

Chapter 10
Trusting others, trusting yourself

Respect yourself, your knowledge and competence

The theme throughout this book has been yourself and nursing, linking in personal development and self-care. This section is talking about respect. If you have completed any of the exercises, the work has been looking at what it means to be a nurse both in terms of characteristics generally and your interpretation.

Respect for yourself is vital so you know how to be respectful to others. A great quote is:- "speak kindly to yourself because you are listening" (Facebook 2016, unattributed to a named person).

Exercise 43. What do you understand by respect? Write down the ways you respect yourself and how other people would know that.

Respect is about putting yourself first and not belittling yourself. Helping and serving people is the core of nursing (Cummings, 2012). Consider it in relation to professional nursing, but also to you as an individual. Another theme I hope comes through this book is that being a nurse is a part of your life, albeit a large part, but it is not your whole life nor who you are.

People talk about work-life balance, however it should be about your life and how your work fits into it. A balanced life is certainly a good aim. It may be that being a nurse is something you love and enjoy but is it your whole purpose in your life? That you have a purpose to do this, that it is the thing that makes you get out of bed in the morning and rush to work and be happy to be there. If that is not what nursing is for you now, or perhaps it was when you started but no longer is, then perhaps you need to re-look at your purpose for nursing and think about what you are doing. Reflect whether it is the best work choice for you at the moment. Respect your feelings and re-purpose yourself. Maybe you need to plan, plan, plan.

In summary, respect yourself in your own right (Dickson, 2015). You have values and principles, adhere to them. Know what you are about, know what your purpose is, know who you are and where you're going with your career. Know what your prize is. How are you going to get the prize? And in your professional life, what is your prize professionally? Where do you want to be? Where is your career and CPD taking you? What is it moving you towards? The option of standing still is not available, because the NMC clearly states that CPD is part of revalidation and re-registration. It was not and should not have been an option with PREP but it was not enforced, therefore nurses could stand still.

Respect for those you care for

The people you are looking after, whether you call them patients, residents, service users, clients or if the people you are looking after are other nurses or members of the multidisciplinary team (MDT), are human beings just like yourself. They have hopes and fears and they can get stressed and distressed and there are many facets to them, they are not just the problem they present with.

This means you have to respect them for who they are. This includes how you speak about them if you are indirectly involved in their care, as a manager or educator. You may or may not have the opportunity to get to know them in full as an individual, but you have the privilege and honour of actually serving and caring for them. For patients this is often when they are at their most vulnerable. Preserving safety for them (NMC, 2015) is the key part. They expect you to be their advocate, they do not expect you to speak about them in a derogatory terms. Therefore, only say things about them that you would say in their hearing.

Remember you have no idea what their background is, you have little concept of what they are dealing with, you do not know what battles they are fighting and you have no idea how it feels to be them. If they are ill or injured and are dependent on healthcare professionals, perhaps for basic intimate personal care they would normal undertake themselves, they may feel frightened and/or vulnerable. Giving respect to people is about prioritising, ensuring you practice effectively and that you showed professionalism because they are trusting you as a nurse to do what is right for them (NMC, 2015). It is important to conduct yourself in a way you would want an another nurse to behave towards you or your loved ones.

Patients' vulnerability may come from a radically altered ability to care for themselves in the way they normally would. If asked to put on unusual clothes, such as a hospital gown, it can be very difficult to stand up for your rights if they feel exposed without their own clothes. Advocacy and preserving safety is also about preserving dignity. Feeling vulnerable may cause someone to become anxious and potentially aggressive. They are going through some form of the grieving process and anger is one of the stages that might manifest (Kűbler-Ross, 2014). Grieving for the loss of person that they were and things they were able to do for themselves before. Aggression may be physical or verbal or both, which necessitates taking action to preserve your own safety and the safety of any of those in the immediate vicinity.

If you are a manager or educator and you are caring for other members of staff, it is about ensuring they do not feel defenceless or helpless by the way in which they are treated by yourself or other staff. Promoting an atmosphere of encouragement and acceptance towards individuals provides a positive environment in which people feel comfortable to work. Preserving safety is about reducing the risk of bullying and/or harassment in the workplace (NMC, 2015).

Students who are new to academic study, nursing or who are returning after a long period away from academic study may feel their lack of knowledge exposes them and renders them vulnerable to failure.

Respect for people's loved ones

Respect for patients' relatives - their family, loved ones, the people who are precious to them and they really care for. These people are often going to be very protective of the patient you are looking after. Omitting to include them and treat them nicely means that they become angry and upset about the way you are doing, or not doing, things for the person they love. They are also potentially going through the grieving process. The manifestation could be verbal or non-verbal anger and again it is about preserving safety (NMC, 2015).

It is also about prioritising people, in terms of recognising the patient is part of an entity since most patients are part of some kind of family, whoever that family might consist of (NMC, 2015). It may be people who are blood/genetic relations, it may be by a formal legal relationship, such as marriage or adoption, or it may be people they have strong connections with because they have known and loved them for a period of time, but the arrangements are informal.

The importance of prioritising relatives may be overlooked in the rush to care for the patient. We may think relatives are a bit of a nuisance because quite frankly they can be outspoken. They are still in their own clothes, they know what they want for the person they love who you are looking after and often they tell staff exactly what they should be doing. It is very easy to judge people as testing or difficult. Our challenge is to manage ourselves and our response to them, to avoid judging them. Conversely, recognise when we are beginning to judge them, and use our professional knowledge and know we can only judge them in terms of risk assessment and in relation to how we can de-escalate situations and hopefully prevent an adverse situation occurring. We can do this by finding out how important these connections are and therefore how much we need to involve the family and friends within the care of the person we are looking after. One of the key things to do is to gain their trust.

The media has reduced trust, by reporting how dreadful hospitals are, how badly behaved nurses and doctors are without balancing it with how many good examples of practice in hospitals and by nurses there are. That has not really helped our cause especially when there are incidences like the Francis report where a whole systems failure was discovered and clearly there were nurses involved. This highlighted to the public they are not necessarily safe in hospitals, which is not what we would expect. Sometimes it is about re-establishing trust and being professional and helping people.

Exercise 44. Write down the skills you already have in developing trust and rapport with people that you meet in your daily work. Note if there is anything extra you need and what would you need to do to acquire it.

Respect for colleagues of the multi-disciplinary team

Working with multi-disciplinary team (MDT) links with Practice Effectively point 8 within the NMC Code of Conduct (NMC, 2015).

Exercise 45. Make notes about the past week and how you have:

- "respected the skills, expertise and contributions of your colleagues, referring matters to them when appropriate" (NMC, 2015).
- effectively maintained communication with colleagues.
- evaluate the quality of your work and that of the team with colleagues.

Working as a nurse and working in the NHS or any kind of healthcare facility/ organisation, is challenging in its own right. We work with colleagues or people who are part of the multidisciplinary team. Again it is about being professional and for us to be able to trust them and that they are able to do their job properly, but also that they can trust us to carry out our role as a nurse correctly and to the best of our ability.

Communication is a core element and again in terms of not judging and being derogatory about people that we work with behind their back. If you are talking about colleagues when they are not present, do not say things that you would not want them to hear.

Use the following table to identify which members of the multidisciplinary team you work with in your area and what you know about their role, what you expect them to be able to do for the people you are all caring for. [These are examples, remove and add as appropriate.]

Being a patient advocate means using the strengths of the multidisciplinary team to ensure that the patient receives the best possible care. Ask members of the MDT to describe what they do for the patient, not just assume that you know.

Multi-disciplinary team members:	Their role	Your expectations of them
Information Technology support		
Community Pharmacist		
General Practitioner		
Physiotherapist		
Occupational therapist		
Operational manager		
Chief Executive Officer		
Learning & Development staff		
Faculty Dean		

Table 10

It may be helpful to show and discuss this table with the multidisciplinary team (MDT) members in order to check whether or not your knowledge and expectations matches the role they should be undertaking. This is part of communication and practising effectively and knowing what each other should be doing (NMC, 2015). It makes it easier to refer appropriately to the correct member of the multidisciplinary team.

Educators may be involved in team teaching with staff who do not have a nursing background, which necessitates them understanding the non-nursing lecturers' role.

Respect for nursing and nurses

Healthcare assistants and nurses carry out nursing duties, but it is only qualified nurses who are legally allowed to call themselves a 'registered nurse'. Only nurses who are actively registered with the NMC are able to practice as nurses. What a privilege to be allowed to use the title 'nurse'. Privileges carry with them obligations and throughout this book it has been emphasised that you have personal responsibility.

Respect for people that we work with within the nursing team is vital, but how often do we hear the expression 'nurses eat their own young'? it is more helpful to be positive about everyone's contribution and look at being non-judgemental. You can use professional judgement, on which to base what you do, whilst respecting the knowledge and expertise of the nurses you come into contact with.

The Code of Conduct (NMC, 2015) demands that we exercise professionalism and trust. It is about trusting other nurses to practice. Professionalism is about guiding nurses and supporting them.

Even if you are a newly qualified nurse and just coming into the nursing team, have respect for yourself because you have knowledge and expertise. It may be that in a given situation you may be the only person that thinks about the correct thing to do for the patient at that point in time - never be afraid to speak up. It maybe that other people just have not thought about it and by speaking up, you might positively affect their life.

We have a duty to enable other nurses and members of the nursing team to practice effectively and to preserve safety while they are doing that. It is about us prioritising not only the patients but nurses as well. How do we help each other and build each other's confidence and encourage each other? If someone is a bit behind with their work, think how we can help them? If, in an education situation, a student nurse does not come for help with their assignment(s), even though you have identified help would benefit them - how can you encourage them and ensure they access tutorial, or the learning and development unit staff's, support? The aim being successfully completion of the course which they are undertaking.

From a managerial aspect, the safety issue is often the one that is paramount, are we preserving the safety of the nurses of the patients or both? If we are not preserving the safety of the nurses, they may feel unimportant and that they are not being respected. How then can we expect them to respect others? Respect and valuing is vital in supporting one another. These are paramount in making sure that patients get looked after correctly. By putting patients first, we may be doing our whole business the wrong way round.

Summary

Nursing: your registration. In order to practise as a nurse, you have to maintain your registration and go through the process of revalidation. You must refer to the NMC revalidation website, which is linked on the website for this book. Exercises in this book should have enabled you to explore some of the issues relating to the revalidation process and I have exhorted you to undertake personal development as well as continuing professional development. Neither are simple on your own and at least one guide is advised.

By knowing and understanding your purpose in life, not just as a nurse, things can become easeful. Know who you are and that being a nurse is simply a part of your life.

Now for the celebration and congratulations! You made it to the end of the book! Wow! That is a great achievement! You are awesome! You believed you could do it and you did!

This is not the end, it is a part of your journey and I am privileged that you have allowed me to travel with you. I would really love to carry on the relationship and to continue to guide and serve you as you travel along your nursing career.

Claire Picton

For updated information and free bonuses, including an extended reference list and relevant website links, go to the website for this book.

www.NurseRevalidationBook.co.uk

See you there!

About the author

Since coming to understand herself better through self-development, particularly with the help and support of Lucie Bradbury and the Damsels in Success Leaders, Claire describes herself thus: "I am me and that is enough for me to be."

In her lifetime she has lived with her family, before moving to London to commence her nurse training. Her many, predominantly, women friends, have kept in touch with her and she with them. She is married and has a son and 2 step-sons, plus step-grandchildren. She is also a member of the Christian family.

In addition to her life experiences, Claire has a wealth of professional experience as: Senior Lecturer; Consultant in Emergency Care Nursing and immediate past Editor of Emergency Nurse journal, plus her current roles as Nurse Consultant Practice Development and Director of both, Damsels in Success Uxbridge and Claire Picton Develops (CPD). All of these enable her to effectively guide and motivate nurses.

For bonuses and new content, plus if you want to use Claire's knowledge and expertise further contact her by visiting:

www.NurseRevalidationBook.co.uk

Made in the USA
Middletown, DE
23 April 2017